Lymphoedema
TAKING CONTROL

BC PUBLISHING
SYDNEY, AUSTRALIA

Lymphoedema

TAKING CONTROL

Professor John Boyages, MD, PhD

BC PUBLISHING
SYDNEY, AUSTRALIA

Lymphoedema: Taking Control

BC Publishing
PO Box 568
Beecroft, NSW 2119, Australia
www.bcpublish.com
bcpublishers@gmail.com

Published in Australia. Written in UK English.

Printed in China through Red Planet Print Management, Sydney

ISBN (POD-standard colour): **978-0-9945874-8-0**
ISBN (POD-premium colour): **978-0-9945874-6-6**

Important: The contents of this book should not be used in place of a visit, call, or consultation with and advice given by your physician, qualified lymphoedema therapist or other healthcare providers. Talk to your doctor or pharmacist before taking any prescription or over-the-counter drugs (including herbal medicines or supplements). You should never disregard professional medical advice or delay seeking it because of something you read in this book or on any website. While every effort has been made to ensure that the material in this book is accurate at the time of publication, discoveries are often made, and treatment practices may ultimately change, update, or invalidate some of the information presented here. Any use of this book is at the reader's discretion. While every effort has been made to ensure the information is accurate, complete, and current, BC Publishing and the author do not guarantee and assume no legal liability or responsibility for the accuracy, currency, or completeness of the information.

Reference to external resources in this publication should not be taken as an endorsement or recommendation of any third-party products or services offered, and the views or recommendations provided by these external resources do not necessarily reflect those of BC Publishing. Note that a healthcare professional should always be consulted regarding your specific situation.

NATIONAL LIBRARY OF AUSTRALIA
A catalogue record for this book is available from the National Library of Australia

Subjects: Lymphoedema; Breast cancer; Arm oedema; Breast oedema; Melanoma; Skin cancer

DEDICATION

To Louise Koelmeyer, who inspired my interest in lymphoedema.

To the incredible team of dedicated lymphoedema clinicians worldwide who work tirelessly to help people navigate this challenging condition.

To my late father, Constantine Steven Boyages, who, with one hand, turned despair into resilience, hope, and optimism.

More Praise for *Lymphoedema: Taking Control*

"With a long-term vision and commitment to strategy focused on helping and supporting patients, John Boyages and I have worked together for years to improve lymphoedema care. This book is an essential part of that mission."

—Associate Professor Louise Koelmeyer, Director of the Australian Lymphoedema Education, Research and Treatment (ALERT) Centre at Macquarie University

"John Boyages is a leader in the field of lymphoedema treatment. His dedication and expertise shine through in this must-read book for patients and healthcare professionals alike."

—Clinical Associate Professor Helen Mackie, Medical Lead of the ALERT Centre at Macquarie University

"John has crafted an extraordinary resource for patients and clinicians dealing with breast cancer-related lymphoedema. His focus on empowering patients with knowledge, practical strategies and the latest research makes this book an invaluable guide."

—Professor Sheila Ridner, Ingram Professor of Nursing at Vanderbilt University School of Nursing

"This comprehensive book on lymphedema offers a modern approach to diagnosis, prevention, and treatment. It is an essential guide for anyone facing lymphoedema or supporting someone through it. John Boyages combines empathy and expertise, providing a clear and compassionate roadmap for understanding and managing this condition. Beyond practical aspects of care, the book addresses the emotional challenges patients face. John's commitment to education and deep understanding make this book an invaluable resource for patients, families, and healthcare providers."

—Professor Alphonse Taghian, Professor of Radiation Oncology at Harvard Medical School and Director of the Lymphedema Research Program at Massachusetts General Hospital

Contents

Foreword 9
About the author 10
Introduction 12

1 UNDERSTANDING THE LYMPHATIC SYSTEM 14
2 WHAT IS LYMPHOEDEMA? 20
3 RISK FACTORS FOR LYMPHOEDEMA 26
4 CLINICAL ASSESSMENT AND TESTS 34
5 EARLY DETECTION AND INTERVENTION 48
6 COMPLEX LYMPHOEDEMA THERAPY 54
7 SKIN CARE AND LYMPHOEDEMA 70
8 ALL ABOUT COMPRESSION GARMENTS 76
9 OTHER LYMPHOEDEMA THERAPIES 90
10 LIPOSUCTION FOR LYMPHOEDEMA 98
11 LYMPHATIC MICROSURGERY 110
12 LYMPHOEDEMA PRECAUTIONS – FACT VS FICTION 118
13 PREVENTION AND TREATMENT OF CELLULITIS 132
14 BREAST OEDEMA 144
15 THE EMOTIONAL SIDE OF LYMPHOEDEMA 156

PATIENT STORIES 96, 97, 106, 107, 116, 142, 162

ENDNOTES
Credits 168
Abbreviations 169
Glossary 170
Useful websites 174
References 177
Index 187

Foreword

Having dedicated over 30 years to the field of lymphoedema management and breast cancer rehabilitation, I am deeply honoured to write this foreword for *Lymphoedema: Taking Control* by Professor John Boyages. This book is a testament to John's unwavering commitment to improving the lives of those affected by lymphoedema.

John and I have collaborated for nearly three decades, first at the Westmead Breast Cancer Institute and then at the Australian Lymphoedema Education, Research and Treatment (ALERT) Centre from 2012. Our shared vision has remained constant: to empower patients with the knowledge and practical tools to manage their lymphoedema effectively. This book is an extension of that vision, offering a comprehensive yet accessible guide for individuals living with or at risk of lymphoedema, as well as their caregivers and healthcare professionals.

Lymphoedema can be a life-changing condition, but it does not have to be faced alone or without support. John's book covers every aspect of lymphoedema care, from assessment and early detection to practical management strategies. It also explores the role of complex lymphoedema therapy and advanced surgical treatment options such as liposuction. Additionally, crucial topics like skin care, the emotional challenges and the unique concerns associated with breast oedema are covered.

What truly sets this book apart is its patient-centred approach. John has always been a visionary and a strong advocate for patients, ensuring that their voices are heard and their needs addressed. This ethos shines through in the book, which presents clear, well-researched information designed to empower readers to take control of their health and well-being. *Lymphoedema: Taking Control* is a reflection of, and testament to, John's expertise, compassion and dedication to the field of lymphoedema management. I highly recommend this book and trust that it will serve as an invaluable resource, providing the guidance and support that patients need to lead fulfilling lives.

Associate Professor Louise Koelmeyer, PhD

Director, ALERT Centre, Faculty of Medicine,
Health & Human Sciences, Macquarie University

About the author

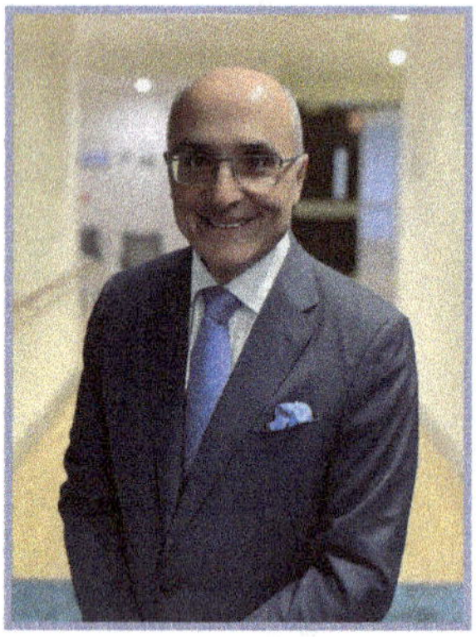

Professor John Boyages, MD, PhD is a cancer specialist with 40 years of experience in breast cancer management. He is a radiation oncologist at Icon Cancer Centre, and founding director and honorary professor of the Australian Lymphoedema Education, Research and Treatment (ALERT) Centre.

Following his fellowship at Harvard Medical School, John was appointed as a specialist radiation oncologist at Westmead Hospital in 1989, and in 1993 he founded Australia's largest free breast screening program in Sydney's west. In 1995, he established and directed the Westmead Breast Cancer Institute, a comprehensive breast cancer program. John established the ALERT lymphoedema program at Macquarie University in 2012.

John has published more than 200 research and clinical articles and is a reviewer for multiple international journals. In 2010, John published his bestselling and award-winning book, *Breast Cancer: Taking Control*, for patients with breast cancer. In 2014, he published *DCIS of the Breast: Taking Control* and *Male Breast Cancer: Taking Control*. In 2021, he continued the series with *Cancer & Vaccinations: Taking Control*.

In addition to his research, John works as a radiation oncologist providing expert care to patients with breast cancer in Sydney. He enjoys spending spare moments with his family and friends, enjoys bushwalking and is learning bridge and oil painting.

In 2017, John was appointed a Member in the General Division of the Order of Australia (AM) for his significant service to medicine.

ACKNOWLEDGEMENTS

I especially want to thank my wife, Dianne, for her patience and support. Thanks also to my beautiful children, Fiona and Peter, son-in-law David and daughter-in-law Lauren, for their ongoing humour, support and understanding. Special mention goes to my beautiful grandchildren: Jack, Anna, Lily, Elsie and Samuel.

Thank you to the experts who reviewed parts of this book, including lymphoedema therapists Melanie Cole, Kate Perkins and Catalina Llanos Escobar.

A special thank you to Cheryl Brunelle, Professor Håkan Brorson, Associate Professor Louise Koelmeyer, Dr Helen Mackie and Professor Sheila Ridner for their critical review of this book.

Introduction

There's no easy way to put this: lymphoedema is very distressing. You may have just got over your treatment, and now you're stuck with a swollen arm as a daily reminder of your cancer journey. Many patients are distressed because while they may be able to hide the scars on their chest, it is tough to hide a swollen arm, particularly when wearing a compression garment.

A national survey from the Australian Lymphoedema Education, Research and Treatment (ALERT) Centre at Macquarie University, showed that patients with lymphoedema reported a significant impact on their work or career, family life, social life, self-image and feelings about themselves (Boyages, 2016). Lymphoedema has been found to have a negative impact on work, finances and sexuality (Boyages, 2017; Winch, 2015). Public insensitivity is also a problem (Kalfa, 2019). One of my patients with lymphoedema, when people repeatedly asked what happened to her arm, would respond that it was from a shark bite as a way of shutting down and diverting the conversation.

If you do get early lymphoedema, there is a possibility that it will not get worse, particularly if you see a therapist and begin active treatment. Stage 1 lymphoedema, where the fluid comes and goes, may still be reversible. Unfortunately, for some patients – particularly those who have had surgery to the armpit followed by chemotherapy and radiotherapy – lymphoedema may appear early, progress, and then become permanent.

It's not easy when a friend or health professional makes patronising comments like "you have to learn to live with it". I've heard others, including doctors, say that lymphoedema is "a small price to pay" for treating cancer, almost as if you should feel grateful!

This book aims to help you or your family member understand the following:

- **The causes and impacts of lymphoedema**
- **How lymphoedema is diagnosed**
- **The advantages of early detection and intervention**
- **How a lymphoedema therapist can help you**
- **Surgical treatment options for lymphoedema**
- **What is fact and what is fiction about lymphoedema**
- **Prevention and treatment of infection (cellulitis)**
- **Swelling of the breast, known as breast oedema**
- **The emotional side of lymphoedema.**

This book applies to men and women with lymphoedema, particularly after cancer treatment to the breast, arm or hand, or those who are at risk of developing lymphoedema. Although this book specifically focuses on the arm, hand and breast, many sections also apply to lymphoedema in other body parts, including the leg. However, most of the research that I reference in this book is related to breast cancer.

Terms that appear in **bold** are defined in the glossary. There is also a section called "Useful websites" at the end of this book, which contains the URLs of any web pages referenced in the text, along with other recommended resources.

1

UNDERSTANDING THE LYMPHATIC SYSTEM

WHAT IS THE LYMPHATIC SYSTEM?

The **lymphatic system** is your body's drainage system, which collects excess fluid from tissues and returns it to the bloodstream. The lymphatic system helps to push nutrients, fluids and immune cells called lymphocytes and **macrophages** into the body's tissues to supply them with food, oxygen, and protection from infections and other diseases.

The lymphatic system removes all the fluids and their contents that leak into the tissues, as well as waste products and bacteria.

A major component of the lymphatic system is the extensive network of thin tubes, called lymphatic vessels, which carry **lymph** around your body. It is this network that connects your arteries, which carry oxygenated blood from the heart to organs and tissues, to your veins, which carry the deoxygenated blood back to the heart and lungs (see **Figure 1.1**).

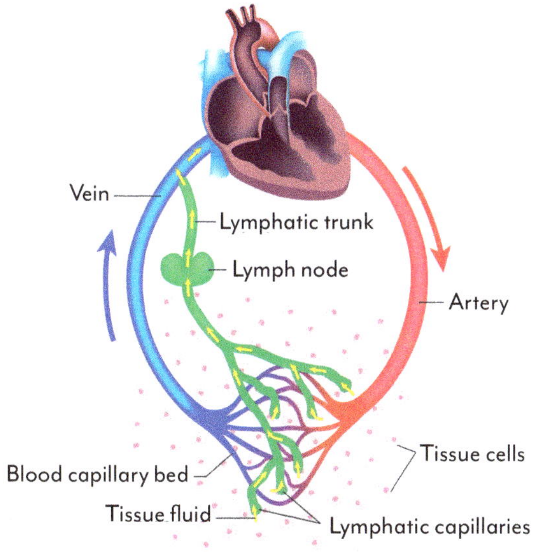

Figure 1.1

The lymphatic capillaries join blood capillaries in the organs and tissues, taking waste products to the lymph node.

Lymphatic vessels connect to your **lymph nodes** (sometimes called lymph glands): small, bean-shaped structures that act as filtration centres, trapping and destroying bugs and abnormal cells. Other lymphatic organs such as the spleen, thymus and tonsils play an essential role in immune function by producing and storing white blood cells to combat infections.

The smallest lymphatic vessels, called **lymphatic capillaries** (also known as initial lymphatics or lymph capillaries), are found in tissues throughout the body. Unlike arteries and veins, these vessels are tiny and do not have any functioning valves. When the pressure in the surrounding fat and tissues increases, lymphatic anchors called filaments pull up the cells lining the lymphatic capillaries, allowing fluid to move through them towards progressively larger lymphatic vessels.

After the fluid (lymph) is filtered by the lymph nodes, most of it empties back into the blood through the largest lymphatic channel in the body, the **thoracic duct**, which connects to a large vein in the lower part of your left neck. Lymph from the right upper body (right arm, face, and part of the right chest) empties into the blood through the right lymphatic duct.

STRUCTURE OF THE LYMPHATIC SYSTEM

The lymphatic capillaries, located throughout the body, originate near blood capillaries and cover your entire body surface. Lymphatic capillaries are tiny channels lined by a single layer of continuous or overlapping cells called **endothelial cells**. Fibres called anchoring filaments connect the lymphatic capillaries to the surrounding tissues.

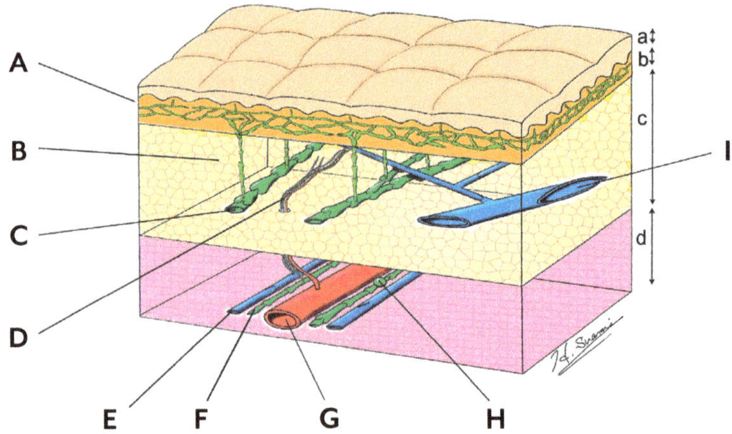

A: Lymphatic capillary, **B**: Precollector, **C**: Superficial lymphatic collector, **D**: Perforating lymphatic vessel and artery, **E**: Deep vein, **F**: Deep lymphatic collector, **G**: Artery, **H**: Interval lymph node, **I**: Superficial vein, a: Epidermis, b: Dermis, c: Fat, d: Muscle.

Figure 1.2

Structure of the lymphatic system. Copyright Hiroo Suami, with permission.

When fluid leaves the blood capillaries into the surrounding tissues, the increased volume and pressure causes the anchoring filaments to open the overlapping endothelial cells. The fluid then moves into the lymphatic system, because pressure is lower in the lymphatic capillaries (see **Figure 1.2A**) than in the surrounding tissue.

The endothelial junctions (spaces that open up between the cells) close once the pressure in the lymphatic capillaries is higher than the tissue pressure outside. This moves the fluid into the precollectors (**Figure 1.2B**), which are larger vessels connecting lymphatic capillaries to the superficial lymphatic collectors (**Figure 1.2C**).

In contrast to the tiny lymphatic capillaries, lymphatic collectors contain valves. The segment between a pair of valves, known as a lymphangion, contracts to transport the fluid upward. Lymphatic collectors transport fluid to the lymph nodes and larger lymphatic trunks that drain into large veins. Lymphatic flow is increased with muscle movement, breathing, and pulsation of the arteries.

There is also a deep lymphatic system with deep lymphatic collectors (**Figure 1.2F**) around the bone, muscle and the more rigid "connective tissue" or **deep fascia** that surrounds them. The superficial and deep lymphatic systems are largely independent, but connections can sometimes occur.

HOW ARE LYMPH NODES CONNECTED TO THE LYMPHATIC VESSELS?

Lymph nodes are classified as "regional" or "interval" according to their location. **Regional lymph nodes** drain lymph from your skin or deeper organs; they are treated by surgery or **radiation**, as cancer cells often spread there first. For example, cancers of the hand, arm or breast can spread to one or more regional lymph nodes in the armpit (**axilla**).

Interval lymph nodes are found in your limbs, and the lymphatic vessels pass through them to the regional lymph nodes. They are sometimes called "in-transit nodes". One example is the epitrochlear node, just above your elbow. This node may be involved with skin cancer, such as melanoma or squamous cell carcinoma (SCC). Other interval lymph nodes in the deep lymphatic system are located along the main arteries in the limbs (**Figure 1.2G–H**).

The first draining regional lymph node (which is usually, but not always, closest to the tumour) is called the **sentinel lymph node**, and it receives multiple lymphatic channels from the area in the body where your cancer started. The sentinel node is a type of "guardian" lymph gland, and it is thought that the lymphatic vessels drain there first before being connected to other lymph nodes. For example, in breast cancer, there are usually one to three sentinel nodes in the axilla draining each breast. Similarly, sentinel nodes can be found in other regions, such as in the groin for cancers of the leg, where they serve the same purpose as the first line of defence in the lymphatic system.

The lymph nodes are very important for immunity. The lymphatic system also includes the tonsils, the thymus (a gland in the upper chest that is larger in childhood) and the spleen (in the upper left abdomen), as well as multiple lymph nodes around the arms, legs, chest and abdomen.

HOW ARE LYMPH NODES ORGANISED IN THE ARMPIT?

The lymph nodes in your armpit (also called the axilla) are known as axillary lymph nodes. **Figure 1.3** shows how the axillary nodes are organised around the pectoralis minor, the muscle underneath the pectoralis major. (Most people call the pectoralis major "the pec", and it is prominent in weightlifters.) There is an average of 25 lymph nodes in three separate areas, or levels, of the axilla. There are approximately 18 lymph nodes in level I, four in level II, and three in level III (Chua and Boyages, 2002).

The levels describe the location of the lymph nodes relative to the pectoralis minor. Level I nodes are found below the muscle, towards the arm; level II nodes are behind the muscle, and level III nodes are above the muscle, towards the collarbone (**Figure 1.3**).

The level III axillary nodes are in the highest point of the armpit, about one inch (2.5cm) from the suprasternal notch, which is the hollow in the top centre of your breastbone. These nodes are also called the infraclavicular nodes, as they sit below your clavicle (collarbone).

The axillary lymph nodes are not the only nodes in this part of the body. There are lymph nodes at the base of your neck above the collarbone, just above the level III axillary nodes. This area is called the **supraclavicular fossa**, or SCF. There are also some lymph nodes between the ribs and the breastbone known as the internal mammary chain (IMC) nodes (**Figure 1.3**).

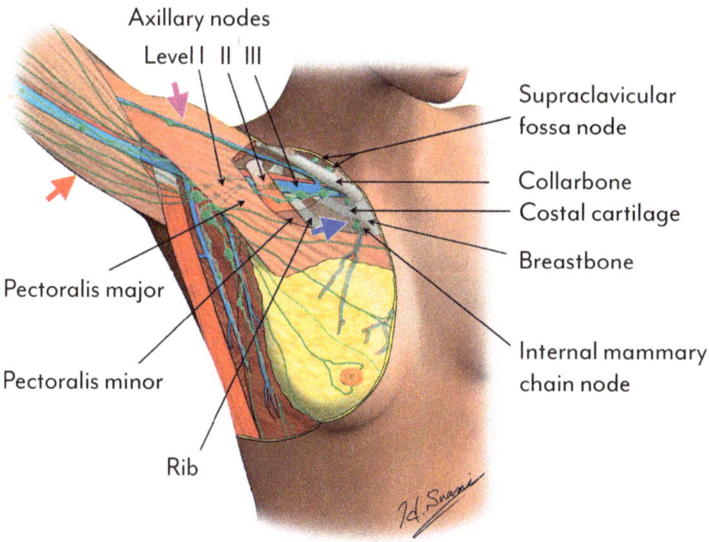

Figure 1.3

There are three groups of lymph nodes draining the arm and chest area – in the armpit (axilla), above the collarbone (supraclavicular fossa) and beside the breastbone (internal mammary chain). Lymphatic vessels drain directly to the axilla (red arrow), bypass the axilla to the lower neck (pink) or drain to the internal mammary chain (blue). Copyright Hiroo Suami, with permission.

2

WHAT IS LYMPHOEDEMA?

WHAT IS LYMPHOEDEMA?

Lymphoedema is an accumulation of lymph in the tissues of your arm, leg, neck, face or other locations, that usually causes swelling. Lymphoedema of the arm is mainly caused by axillary treatment of breast or other cancers, which then causes damage to the lymphatic system. Although lymphoedema can develop at any time after cancer treatment, it usually starts in the first few years after treatment.

Having surgery in your axilla increases the risk of scarring and what we call "back pressure". It's a bit like the difference between a fast-flowing river and a slow-flowing river that is blocked by rocks. The blocked river backs up, and the water is often murkier than that of a fast-flowing river. **Oedema** can also occur in your breast if you've had breast conservation; this is discussed further in **Chapter 14**, Breast Oedema.

Professor Sheila Ridner from Vanderbilt University, a world expert on lymphoedema, emphasised in her review of this book that lymphoedema is a symptom and not a disease. It is the result of increasing disruption of the lymphatic vessels described in **Chapter 1**, Understanding the Lymphatic System. In a highly cited publication written as part of her PhD thesis, Professor Ridner identified that swelling is only part of the picture. Women treated for lymphoedema experienced a cluster of symptoms, consisting of altered limb sensation, loss of confidence, decreased physical activity, fatigue and psychological distress (Ridner, 2005). So, managing lymphoedema is not as simple as getting a diagnosis and being prescribed a fluid tablet. It is important to understand the physiological, physical and psychological dimensions of the condition.

If lymphoedema does occur, its onset is usually subtle and not very noticeable. You may only have some unusual sensations at first, such as tingling in your arm. Other early symptoms of lymphoedema include heaviness, aching and fluctuating swelling, often starting just below the elbow, and sometimes in the hands or fingers – for example, your rings might start to feel tight. Later symptoms include swelling in the forearm, upper arm, or your whole arm. These symptoms may initially settle overnight but can become permanent when more advanced. However, it can progress, and lymphoedema that becomes moderate or severe can affect your function.

Thinking back to the blocked river, imagine what happens when it rains, adding extra water: the river overflows its banks and floods the surrounding fields. Similarly, a blocked or slow-flowing river becomes polluted over time. The same process can happen in your arm or breast when an infection occurs. The volume of lymphatic fluid increases, and it can seep into the soft tissues of your arm, leading to swelling and discomfort.

A severe complication of lymphoedema is cellulitis, an infection of the lymphatic fluid that can spread quickly. This requires urgent antibiotic treatment. If you notice any signs of infection, such as redness, warmth or pain in the affected area, see your doctor immediately to start treatment. Cellulitis may, in fact, be the first sign that you have lymphoedema. Professor Ridner notes that she has had numerous patients report going to bed "fine" and waking up with a hot, aching, swollen arm, which is unresponsive to antibiotics, as their first experience with lymphoedema. For more information, see **Chapter 13**, Prevention and Treatment of Cellulitis.

WHEN CAN LYMPHOEDEMA OCCUR?

Eighty percent of the time, lymphoedema develops in the first 12 to 18 months after surgery. However, the risk of lymphoedema is ongoing and can persist for years after treatment. Recent evidence has found that early detection and intervention may reduce the long-term development of irreversible **chronic lymphoedema** (Ridner, 2019). Technology such as **bioimpedance spectroscopy (BIS)** may detect lymphoedema up to ten months earlier than the previous "gold standard" of using a tape measure to measure limb girth. If you are concerned, a bioimpedance measurement may be helpful to detect lymphoedema before it is visible to you or your doctor (see **Chapter 5**, Early Detection and Intervention).

HOW IS LYMPHOEDEMA CLASSIFIED?

The International Society of Lymphology has classified lymphoedema in various stages of severity **(Figure 2.1)**, as follows:

- Stage 0: A "subclinical" condition where swelling is not yet evident, but subtle symptoms may be present. It may exist for months or years before overt swelling occurs **(see Chapter 5**, Early Detection and Intervention).
- Stage 1: Early accumulation of tissue fluid, which subsides with elevation of your arm. **Pitting** may occur. This means if you

press into the swelling with your thumb for about a minute, your thumb leaves an indentation.

- Stage 2A: Increased accumulation of tissue fluid, and swelling that is rarely reduced by elevating the arm. It can still be pitted or indented.
- Stage 2B: At this stage, the body responds to the fluid by depositing excess fat in the affected area, leading to scarring (**fibrosis**). This means pitting does not easily occur.
- Stage 3: This stage is sometimes called "elephantiasis", as the arm may look like the trunk of an elephant, with wrinkling, thickened and pigmented skin and warty overgrowths. There is no pitting.

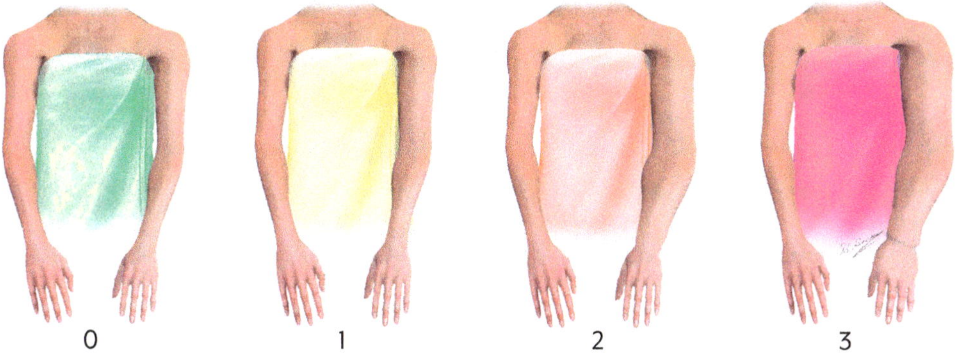

Figure 2.1

The stages of lymphoedema, according to the International Society of Lymphology (ISL, 2023). Copyright Hiroo Suami, with permission.

WHAT IS THE RELATIONSHIP BETWEEN LYMPHOEDEMA AND FAT?

Undoubtedly, the lymphatic system and body fat are intimately related. We know that lymphatic vessels are present within the fat (called **adipose tissue**), and lymph nodes are also surrounded by body fat.

Lymphoedema, however, is far more complicated. When lymphatic fluid slows down or leaks into the surrounding tissue, this protein-rich fluid causes inflammation. Repair cells from the immune system called macrophages and phagocytes appear, and scarring or fibrosis develops. The skin can become thickened.

This inflammation is thought to stimulate adipose stem cells to grow and deposit more fat into the arm. We found this in a Macquarie University study comparing **magnetic resonance imaging (MRI)** scans before and after **liposuction** (Sen and Boyages, 2018) (**Figure 2.2**).

However, it is still essential to try compression, because our MRI studies have found that there is usually surrounding fluid under the skin and in the deep tissues with lymphoedema, and this can still be helped with massage, compression garments or compression devices.

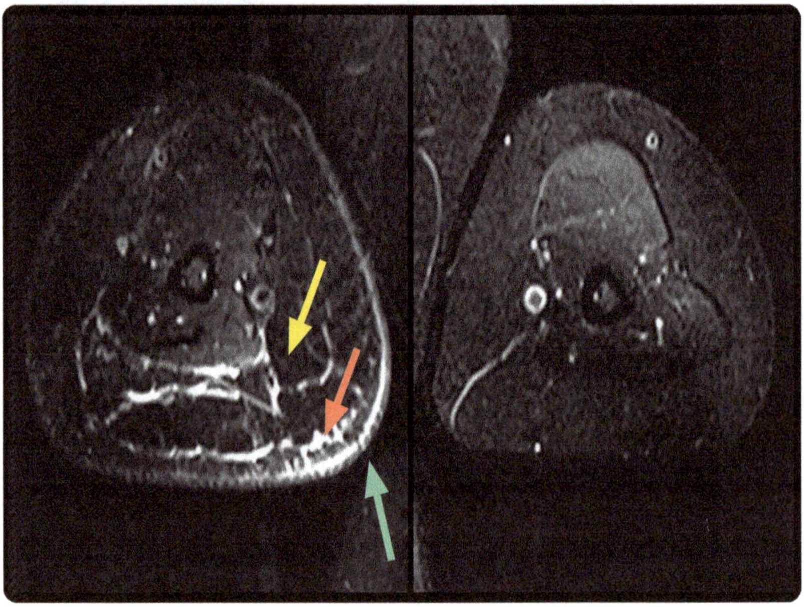

Figure 2.2

MRI cross-section scan of an arm with lymphoedema (left) and without lymphoedema (right). The arm with lymphoedema has increased fat (yellow arrow), lymphatic fluid (red), and thickened skin (green).

In the earlier stages of lymphoedema (stage 1 or 2A), pitting will occur, meaning the fluid can be depressed with pressure from your thumb: when you press for about a minute, your thumb leaves an indentation in the skin (**Figure 2.3A**). This is like getting indentations from your socks when you have swollen feet. The presence of pitting means there is fluid (lymph) accumulating in your arm that can be helped with therapy. If there is no indentation, it means that the lymphoedema has progressed to stage 2B or

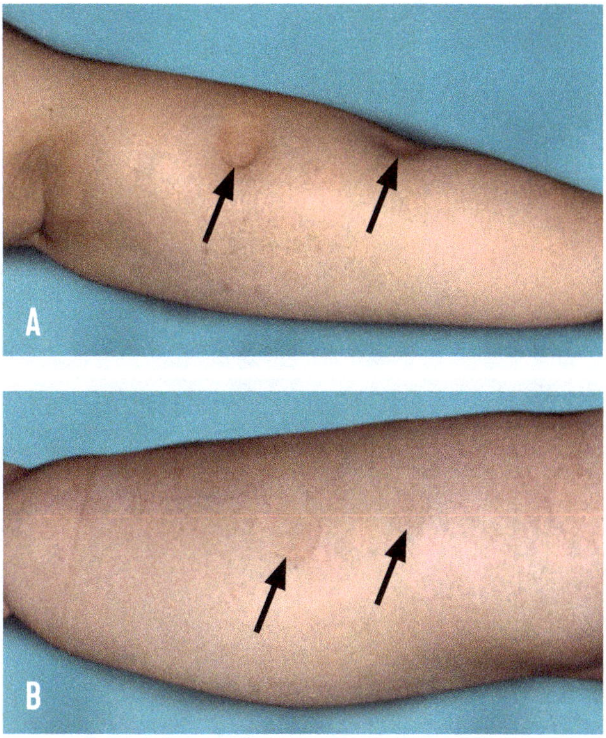

Figure 2.3

The "pitting test": press your thumb into the swollen area for at least a minute and see if you can cause an indentation (A), showing the presence of fluid; minimal indentation (B) shows fat and scarring (fibrosis). Copyright Håkan Brorson, with permission.

stage 3, with fatty deposition and fibrosis, which is more difficult to treat with therapy (**Figure 2.3B**).

For now, it is essential to know that as lymphoedema advances in stages, and as more fat is deposited and fibrosis occurs, it can be more challenging to treat. Compression garments and massage will still provide some symptom relief and support, but their impact may be less obvious.

Therapy options for lymphoedema in the early stages are discussed further in **Chapter 6**, Complex Lymphoedema Therapy.

3

RISK FACTORS FOR LYMPHOEDEMA

AM I AT INCREASED RISK OF LYMPHOEDEMA?

The most important factors that increase the risk of lymphoedema include:

- Extent of surgery and whether you've had a lymph node dissection
- Radiation therapy to lymph nodes in your armpit (axilla) or above the collarbone (supraclavicular fossa)
- Infection or accumulation of fluid lumps (**seroma**) after your surgery
- Being overweight (body mass index [BMI] over 25) or obese (BMI over 30)
- Immobility
- Treatment with certain chemotherapy drugs (taxanes).

Your race or ethnicity may also be a factor. Recent research by Heller (2024) found that the rate of developing lymphoedema after axillary dissection was higher in Black women (31%) and Hispanic women (27%) compared to White women (17%) and Asian women (15%). Asian, Black and Hispanic women also reported lower quality of life scores in their follow-up after surgery. Living in a rural location has also been associated with an increased risk of lymphoedema after breast cancer treatment, possibly due to poorer access to healthcare (Koelmeyer, 2022).

WHAT IS MY LYMPHOEDEMA RISK AFTER AXILLARY SURGERY OR RADIATION?

One of the major risk factors for arm lymphoedema is having surgery to your axilla. This could be a biopsy of one or two of your lymph nodes (sentinel node biopsy), or an **axillary lymph node dissection** (ALND), which is an operation to remove multiple lymph nodes from under your arm. A study at Harvard's Massachusetts General Hospital (MGH) found that the five-year risk of swelling to the arm, as detected by a **perometer**, increased with the amount of treatment to the axilla (Naoum, 2020). This is shown in **Table 3.1** on the following page.

This study carefully compared the volume of the affected arm to that of the unaffected arm, which acted as a "control". Lymphoedema was defined as an increase in arm volume of 10% or more compared to the unaffected arm, and compared to the preoperative baseline, at least three months after surgery.

TREATMENT TO THE AXILLA	Number of patients	5-year risk of lymphoedema
Sentinel node biopsy (SNB)	1,340	8%
SNB + radiation to the lymph nodes	121	11%
Axillary lymph node dissection (ALND)	91	25%
ALND + radiation	263	30%

Table 3.1

The risk of chronic lymphoedema occurring within five years of treatment to the axilla (Naoum, 2020).

This long-term study followed more than 1,800 lymphoedema patients over 13 years. It showed that as the amount of treatment to the axilla increased, so did the risk of developing chronic lymphoedema. A major finding of the study was that the main risk factor for developing lymphoedema was axillary dissection, rather than radiation.

Another Macquarie University study that we conducted with Vanderbilt University was called the PREVENT study, which followed 879 patients with breast cancer who received different types of treatment (Ridner, 2022).

The study was investigating how many patients would develop persistent or chronic lymphoedema requiring **complex lymphoedema therapy (CLT)** within three years of axillary treatment, by close monitoring with either a tape measure or bioimpedance spectroscopy. CLT is discussed in **Chapter 6**, Complex Lymphoedema Therapy.

After an average follow-up time of three years, 69 of the 881 patients (7.8%) had developed chronic lymphoedema. For the patients whose measurements were done by tape measure, almost 10% developed lymphoedema requiring a compression garment, compared to only 6% for those who had their measurements done with bioimpedance spectroscopy. The risk of chronic lymphoedema by surgery or radiation to the axilla is shown in **Table 3.2**.

By the end of three years, the rates of developing chronic lymphoedema were 4% after sentinel node biopsy and 26% after ALND, whether or not radiation was given. That is, having radiation in addition to lymph node surgery did not greatly increase the risk over and above the risk from surgery to the axilla; this is consistent with the findings of the MGH study (Naoum, 2020) described above. However, we did find that the risk of

TREATMENT TO THE AXILLA	Number of patients	2-year risk of lymphoedema
Sentinel node biopsy (SNB)	651	2%
SNB + radiation to the lymph nodes	58	3%
Axillary lymph node dissection (ALND)	85	17%
ALND + radiation	87	24%

Table 3.2

The risk of chronic lymphoedema occurring by the extent of treatment to the axilla (Boyages, 2023).

lymphoedema increased by 3–4% when radiation was given to lymph nodes in the supraclavicular fossa (see **Figure 1.3** for a diagram showing the location of these nodes).

Both PREVENT and the MGH study involved prospective surveillance – that is, screening patients carefully for lymphoedema after their cancer treatment, because of the known risk. Lymphoedema rates are likely to be much higher without active surveillance, reaching rates as high as 35% (Koelmeyer, 2019, Soran, 2014). (See also **Chapter 5**, Early Detection and Intervention.)

OTHER RISK FACTORS FOR LYMPHOEDEMA

The PREVENT study found that the risk of lymphoedema was higher in patients who were overweight or obese, lived in a rural location, received taxane-based chemotherapy or had three or more lymph nodes removed from their axilla.

In a joint study with the Western Sydney University, we surveyed over 200 women who were previously treated for breast cancer (Boyages, 2022). We found that 51% of women with lymphoedema were overweight or obese (with a BMI of 25 or more) at the time of their breast cancer diagnosis. This contrasts with 36% of women without lymphoedema. The study also revealed that 21% of women with lymphoedema were classified as obese (BMI ≥30), compared to just 12% of those without the condition.

If you are overweight or obese, achieving and maintaining a healthy weight can help reduce your risk of developing lymphoedema. By focusing on weight management as part of a broader approach to lymphoedema prevention, you can take proactive steps to protect your health.

WHAT IS CORDING, AND DOES IT CAUSE LYMPHOEDEMA?

Cording, also known as axillary web syndrome (AWS), can develop following surgical procedures like ALND or sentinel node biopsy. Cording appears as a visible and palpable cord-like structure beneath the skin, resembling guitar strings or a piece of thin rope. It occurs typically in the axillary (armpit) region, extending down the inner arm to the elbow and sometimes down the inner forearm (**Figure 3.1**).

Cording was first described by Ferrandez and Serin (1996) as being caused by lymphatic inflammation and clotting of the lymphatic fluid. Moskovitz (2001), from the University of Washington, biopsied four patients and found that two patients had dilated lymphatic vessels (including one patient with a fibrous clot inside the vessel) and three patients had clots inside a small vein in various stages of reopening. A recent study examined small tissue samples taken from cording in seven patients. The study found that three of the cord samples were from lymphatic vessels. In one of these samples, the vessel was blocked by a clot that had become firm over time (Johansson, 2020).

Cording can cause discomfort in everyday tasks such as placing something on a shelf, putting on a bra that clips at the back, drying your back with a towel, and cleaning above shoulder height (Brunelle, 2020). The cording becomes visible or palpable and painful when the shoulder is lifted or raised sideways (abducted).

A recent Harvard study of over 1000 patients found that three in ten women with breast cancer reported cording in the axilla or the breast area. Cording in the axilla occurred in one in four patients (Brunelle, 2020). Cording was more common in patients who were under 55 and were treated with a mastectomy, an axillary lymph node dissection, chemotherapy or radiation to the lymph nodes.

Another study found that cording occurred less often after a sentinel node biopsy (20%) than an axillary dissection (72%). For people who had cording after an axillary dissection, there was a one in four chance that the cord would reach down to the forearm. On the other hand, none of the patients with cording after a sentinel node biopsy had the cord extend this far down their arm (Leidenius, 2003).

In a Spanish study by Torres Lacomba (2009), physiotherapists examined 270 patients for cording at five visits over the first year after treatment.

They found the incidence of cording was nearly one in two patients (48%). Symptoms included tenderness (61%), aching (61%), and firmness/tightness (60%). Most cases of cording occurred mainly in the first two weeks after surgery; there were three instances of cording occurring three to seven months after surgery, once chemotherapy and radiation were completed. Reassuringly, the cording had resolved three months after surgery for most patients.

One **systematic review** could not confirm a definite link between cording and lymphoedema (Yeung, 2015). However, Brunelle (2020) found that patients with cording were more than twice as likely to develop lymphoedema, compared to patients without cording. This study suggests that cording should be considered a potential risk factor when screening for lymphoedema after breast cancer treatment.

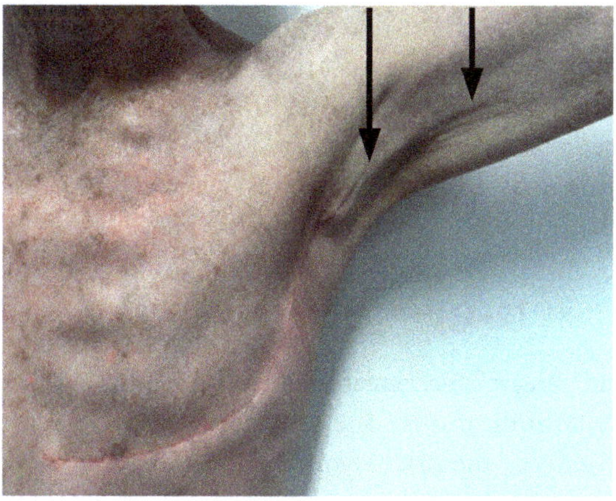

Figure 3.1

Typical cording occurring about eight weeks after axillary surgery.

Treatment options for cording

There are currently no evidence-based guidelines or clinical trials related to cording, so the usual treatment approach for this condition is to explore different options with your physiotherapist or healthcare provider and see what works for you. There are various approaches to treating cording, including therapy techniques such as gentle stretching exercises, myofascial release, deeper massage and cupping to enhance flexibility and reduce tension. You may find that a hot compress helps to ease the inflammation, although you need to be careful to protect your skin, as you may have altered sensation under your armpit after surgery. Take short-term paracetamol or anti-inflammatories to ease the pain and tenderness from cording.

Some therapists use laser therapy or even advise a compression garment to treat cording. If you search for "cording" or "axillary web syndrome" on YouTube, you will find many therapists providing sensible advice about this condition. However, it is important to always seek the advice of an experienced and accredited lymphoedema therapist to treat your cording.

Cording of the breast – Mondor's disease

Mondor's disease is a rare condition caused by inflammation or temporary clotting of veins close to the skin's surface. First described by surgeon Henri Mondor (1939), this condition commonly affects the chest, abdomen, or breast region, leading to visible and often painful cord-like structures that can be easily felt beneath the skin (**Figure 3.2**). In many ways, the bands are similar to cording, and I suspect that some cases result from lymphatic obstruction. While Mondor's disease often resolves without treatment, medical attention may be necessary and involve paracetamol, anti-inflammatories, massage, laser therapy and, more rarely, blood-thinning medication such as aspirin to prevent further blood clots.

PERSONALISING TREATMENT TO PREVENT LYMPHOEDEMA

Over the years, breast cancer treatment has been adjusted ("de-escalated") to minimise complications. The sentinel node biopsy procedure has significantly reduced the risk of lymphoedema in many parts of the body. In the past, when a patient had a small amount of disease in one or two sentinel nodes, we would surgically dissect the axilla. Today, we typically do a sentinel node biopsy followed by radiation; this has the same success rate as an axillary dissection, with a much lower risk of arm swelling. I know some surgeons who are reluctant to do more than a sentinel node biopsy for obese or overweight patients.

For some patients, it's possible to reduce the amount of radiation by not treating the supraclavicular fossa, and this also reduces the risk of lymphoedema. Advanced radiation techniques, such as intensity modulated radiation therapy (IMRT) or volumetric modulated arc therapy (VMAT), can target cancer cells more precisely while sparing healthy tissues and lymphatic structures.

If you have breast cancer on the same side as your dominant arm, and you rely on your arm for work, it may be worth talking to your doctor about the options for treating the lymph nodes surrounding your cancer. It may be possible to customise your treatment to minimise the risk of developing lymphoedema in your dominant arm.

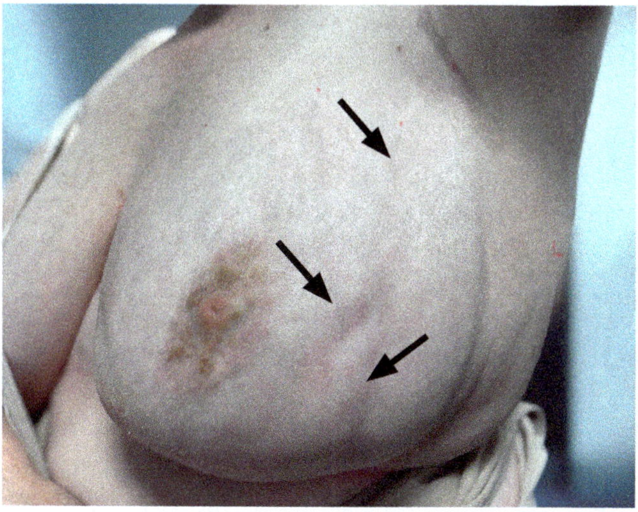

Figure 3.2
Typical cording of the breast (Mondor's disease).

4

CLINICAL ASSESSMENT AND TESTS

The tests used to monitor or screen for lymphoedema can vary depending on where you are receiving care. In some places, your health professional might only use a tape measure, while advanced lymphoedema centres may offer an array of tests, including experimental research devices. Any assessment, even a simple arm circumference measurement, is better than none. As in many areas of medicine, there is no one perfect solution. While experts like Vargo (2024) have reviewed the strengths and weaknesses of various tests, the important thing to remember is that not every test is necessary. The approach should be tailored to your unique situation and will depend on the experience of your healthcare team.

PATIENT HISTORY

The most important part of lymphoedema management is a thorough and holistic assessment. Your healthcare provider should take a full medical history before performing a clinical examination, objective measurements or other tests. During this consultation, several key areas will be explored, as outlined below and on next page.

Social history

A discussion of your lifestyle, who lives at home with you, your occupation and life roles, level of physical activity and function. As health professionals, we always ask about smoking and alcohol consumption. Smoking can impair circulation and your body's ability to heal, and excessive alcohol can cause or worsen swelling and reduce your immunity, potentially increasing the risk of infection (Cavezzi, 2019). These factors can impact both the development of lymphoedema and its day-to-day management.

Medical history

A detailed history of your cancer diagnosis and treatment, such as surgery, chemotherapy or radiotherapy, with particular attention to any involvement or treatment of the lymph nodes. Other past or current illnesses will be reviewed, and any medications you are currently taking, including those prescribed for other conditions such as diabetes, arthritis or past shoulder surgery.

Precipitating factors

Enquiry into any other factors that may have contributed to your lymphoedema, such as infections, trauma or prolonged immobility.

Family history

An assessment of any family history of lymphoedema to identify possible genetic links. It is essential to determine whether you have **primary lymphoedema** (an inherited condition) or **secondary lymphoedema** (related to cancer treatment, trauma or other causes).

Lymphoedema details

Information such as when you first noticed the swelling, its location (e.g., arms, legs, chest) and any associated symptoms like tingling, swelling, heaviness, pain, tightness or limited mobility. Previous episodes of cellulitis or other infections will also be discussed.

Emotional and psychological impact

An exploration of how lymphoedema has affected your emotional wellbeing, daily activities and physical functioning. Any experiences of anxiety, stress or frustration will be considered.

Current management

Details on any treatments you have already tried, including use of compression garments, and how effective they have been.

Personal goals

A discussion of your personal goals for treatment, such as reducing swelling, improving mobility, preventing future complications, or becoming better informed about lymphoedema.

CLINICAL EXAMINATION

First impressions

When I examine a patient with breast cancer, the first thing I do, with the patient sitting up and facing me, is to examine their hands. I look for swelling that fills up the space between the tendons on the back of their hands. Most patients wear rings, so I check to see if their rings are tight or fingers are swollen, comparing both sides to see if the treated side is different to the untreated side.

You can also do this for yourself: look at the back of your hand and stretch out your fingers. You should be able to see your tendons (**Figure 4.1**, green arrow). Now look at the depressions between the tendons, (red arrow). If there is any swelling in the hand, these depressions will be less visible.

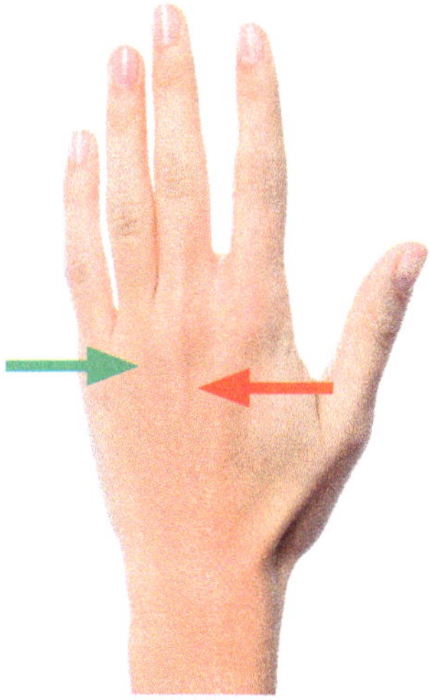

Figure 4.1

The normal back of the hand, showing the tendons (green arrow) and the spaces between (red arrow), which are visible when the hand is not swollen.

I then look at the patient's arms to see if there is any obvious difference in arm circumference between the treated side (i.e. where the patient has undergone surgery or radiation) and the untreated side. **Figure 4.2** shows a patient with visible lymphoedema. The red arrow shows swelling in the back of the hand, which has made the depressions between the tendons disappear. The blue arrow shows indentation caused by a compression garment that has just been removed. The green arrow shows one of the most common locations where lymphoedema swelling first appears. This is where I have tested to see if the oedema was "pitting".

To test for pitting, I usually press my thumb into the outer part of forearm just below the elbow region for at least one minute. If my thumb leaves a depression, there is obvious lymphoedema (**Figure 4.2**, green arrow). This is stage 1 or 2A lymphoedema. If there is swelling in the arm but my thumb leaves no indentation, it means that the lymphoedema has progressed to fatty deposition and scarring (fibrosis) as seen in stage 2B or 3. (See **Figure 2.1** for more about the different stages of lymphoedema.)

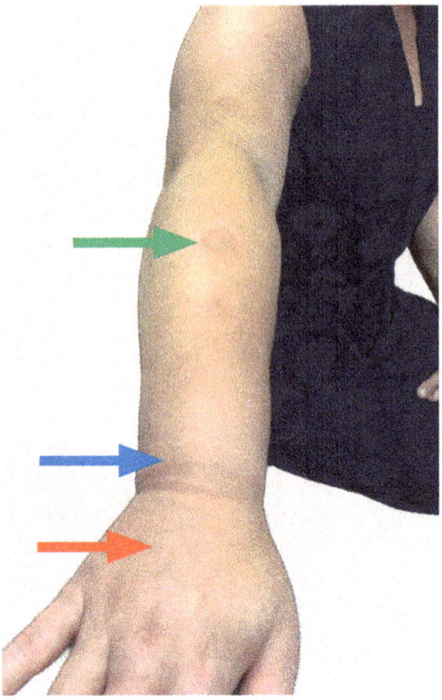

Figure 4.2

A patient presenting with moderate (stage 2A) lymphoedema in the right arm. The red arrow indicates a reduced space between the tendons on the back of the hand. The blue arrow shows indentations from a recently removed compression garment. The green arrow highlights a positive pitting test on the forearm near the elbow, which is one of the most commonly affected areas.

Stemmer's sign

Stemmer's sign is another clinical indicator that can be used to diagnose lymphoedema. It is considered positive when the skin on the top of the index finger or the second toe cannot be easily pinched and lifted. In lymphoedema, the skin in this area becomes thickened and fibrotic, making it difficult to grasp between the fingers (Stemmer, 1976). Realistically, this simple test can be done in any part of the body where lymphoedema is suspected (see **Figure 4.3**).

A positive Stemmer's sign is often one of the early indicators of lymphoedema and can be particularly useful in distinguishing lymphoedema from other causes of swelling. You can try it on yourself over an area where your skin feels different, or where you have possible or confirmed lymphoedema, including the breast. Ask your therapist to show you how to do it. As Professor Håkan Brorson noted on reviewing this book, a negative Stemmer's sign does not rule out lymphoedema, but a positive Stemmer's sign is always evidence of lymphoedema.

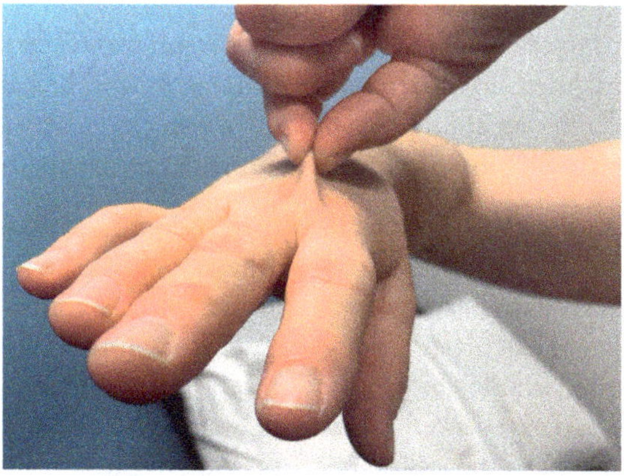

Figure 4.3

Pinching the skin to check for Stemmer's sign. If the skin is thickened and difficult to grasp, it indicates lymphoedema (positive Stemmer's sign). In this patient, the skin is easily lifted, so Stemmer's sign is negative.

TESTS FOR LYMPHOEDEMA

Tape measurements

In the early 1980s, I was trained to use a simple tape measure to take circumference measurements when diagnosing lymphoedema. The degree of lymphoedema was arbitrarily divided into minimal, moderate and severe, based on the difference between the circumference of the arms (treated and untreated), measured at 10cm above and below the bony point of the elbow. A difference in circumference of 2cm or less was minimal, 2.1–4cm was considered moderate, and over 4cm was severe lymphoedema (Boyages, 1988).

Today, with more lymphoedema therapists available, more formal measurements can be taken. Tape measures are still a helpful tool for assessment, but are used with stricter criteria. While measuring limb circumference with a tape measure is quick and simple, it is prone to variations between different readers (known as inter-observer variation) or the same reader (intra-observer variation) (Armer, 2005).

In 2006, when I was the director of the Westmead Breast Cancer Institute, we evaluated the effectiveness of using a tape measure to derive arm volume in patients with and without lymphoedema following breast cancer surgery. We measured the circumference at 10cm intervals from wrist to shoulder, then used this to calculate the volume. This result was compared with the "gold standard" method of water displacement, where the hand and then the arm and hand were submerged in a tub of water to compare the amount of water displaced by the affected arm compared to the unaffected arm.

Both methods showed strong reliability, meaning they produced similar results across different testers, although the circumference measurements slightly overestimated arm volumes compared to water displacement. Arm volume was calculated by adding up the volumes of several small "truncated cone" sections measured along the arm at certain points. This circumference-derived method provided an accurate estimate of arm volume compared to the less practical method of putting a patient's arm in a tub of water (Taylor, 2006).

In the PREVENT trial, we used a similar technique, measuring every 10cm up the arm with a tape measure and then using an equation to determine the arm volume. This volume was then compared to the unaffected arm (Ridner, 2022). Comparing your arm volume on both sides is very important. This is because changes in volume can occur simply because one arm is dominant (right- or left-handed), you've put on weight, or you've lost or gained muscle mass after cancer treatment. It is also extremely helpful to have a baseline measurement for comparison, so ask your treatment team about having both arms measured before you start treatment or have surgery.

The diagram below shows, in simple terms, that arm volume is determined by muscle, fat and lymphatic fluid. An increase in volume can occur due

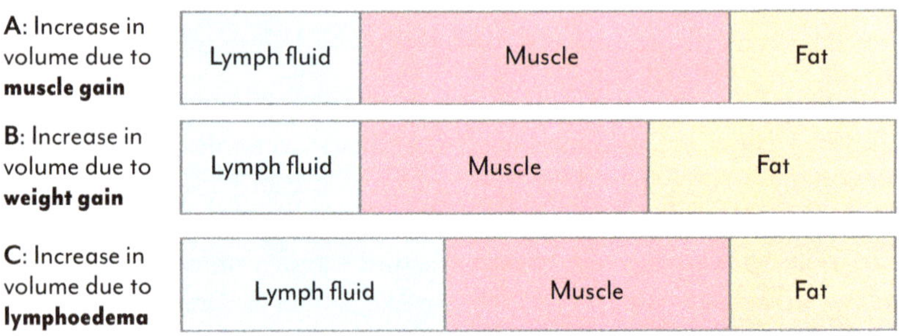

Figure 4.4

Your arm can be thought of as having three compartments that fluctuate in volume. Increases in muscle, fat or lymphatic fluid can change your arm's shape, circumference or volume. Using tape measurements for circumference alone will not be as accurate as volume measurements or bioimpedance spectroscopy.

to an increase in muscle (**Figure 4.4A**) – this muscle mass may be from exercise, or it could be caused by the added heaviness of an arm with lymphoedema (Brorson, 2009). Increased volume can also be due to an increase in fat in your arms (**Figure 4.4B**) or an increase in lymph fluid in the surrounding tissues (**Figure 4.4C**). This is one of the downsides of monitoring for lymphoedema using circumference and volume measures alone, unless there are strict measuring criteria set and both sides are closely compared.

Perometry

A perometer is a harmless infrared measuring device that calculates arm, body or leg volume (**Figure 4.5**). The device measures the circumference and contour of a body part, taking measurements approximately every 5mm, and using these to determine the volume. We have used perometry for many years, initially at the Westmead Breast Cancer Institute and then at the ALERT Centre. A perometer is a quick but costly piece of equipment that also takes up a lot of floor space. My colleague at the Massachusetts General Hospital, Professor Alphonse Taghian, has used perometry to conduct world-leading research on the incidence of lymphoedema after surgery and radiation (Naoum, 2020).

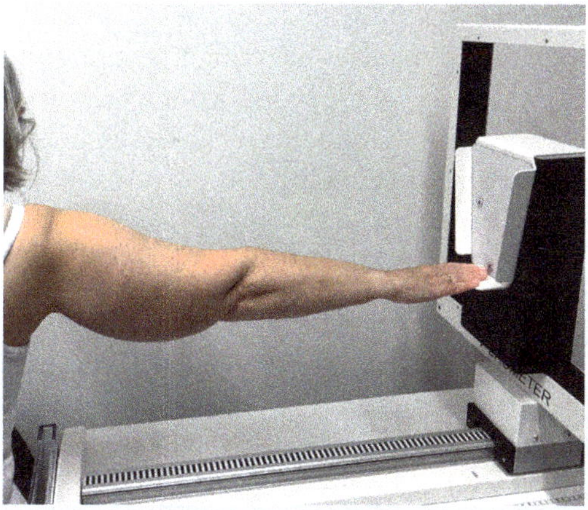

Figure 4.5

A perometer can accurately measure arm or leg volume by taking multiple circumference measurements of the limb in 4.7mm intervals to calculate the volume.
The square frame at the top of the picture moves across your arm in seconds.
There is no radiation and no complications.

Bioimpedance spectroscopy

Bioimpedance spectroscopy is a valuable tool for detecting lymphoedema before you or your healthcare professional can see it. It may also be helpful if you have already been diagnosed with lymphoedema. This non-invasive test works by measuring the resistance of your body tissues to a small, safe electrical current, which helps assess the fluid levels in your affected limb.

Measuring with bioimpedance spectroscopy gives what is known as an L-Dex (lymphoedema index) score. Comparing the L-Dex scores of your affected and unaffected sides allows your healthcare team to monitor the progression of your lymphoedema, evaluate how well your treatment is working, and make informed decisions about your ongoing care. Bioimpedance is particularly useful because it provides an objective measurement to complement physical examination, and the volume tests described above. It's a quick test that gives a visual representation of the fluid levels in your arm or leg, so you can see how the limb is responding to treatment (see **Figure 5.2**). I will look more closely at bioimpedance spectroscopy in **Chapter 5**, Early Detection and Intervention.

Nuclear studies – lymphoscintigraphy

If you had a sentinel node biopsy as part of your cancer treatment, you may have already had a lymphoscintigram. This nuclear imaging procedure uses the same equipment but involves injecting tiny amounts of radioactive particles into the web spaces at the base of your fingers, toes or other areas affected by lymphoedema. Although the procedure uses a small amount of radioactive material, it is very safe, as the levels are extremely low and pose no risk to your health.

This injected radioactive material gives off energy as gamma rays, which can be detected by a gamma camera. The camera produces images that reflect the amount of radiotracer absorbed throughout your lymphatic system. The test can take up to two hours, and the injections can sting a little at first. The pictures can be challenging to interpret, but they will show if your lymphatic system has taken up the radioactive dye.

For the patient in **Figure 4.6**, the images have been taken 30 minutes after injection of the tracer. On the right side, the dye has moved rapidly up the arm to the axilla, showing a normal right lymph node (red arrow).

By comparison, on the patient's left-hand side there is no activity in the lymph node, but the dye is spreading around the skin – this is known as **dermal backflow**. An advantage of lymphoscintigraphy over indocyanine green (ICG) fluorescent lymphography (discussed below) is that you can see if lymph nodes deeper in the body are functioning and take up the radioactive dye. The ICG dye only scans about 1cm beneath the skin; it shows your lymphatic circulation, but not the underlying lymph nodes or deeper lymphatic vessels.

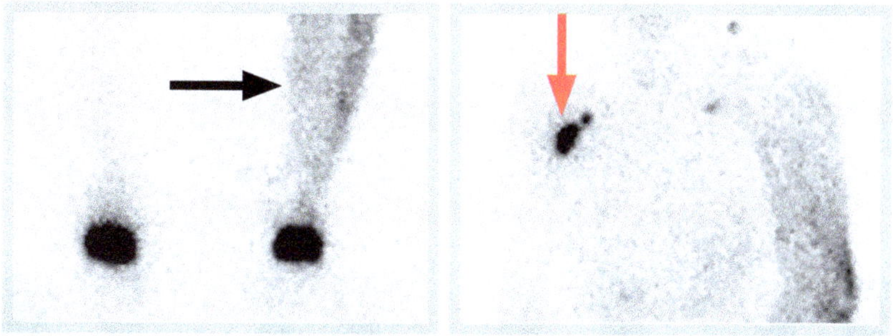

Figure 4.6
Lymphoscintigram for a patient with left-sided lymphoedema after breast cancer treatment. The red arrow shows a normal lymph node in the right axilla. The left side shows uptake around the skin consistent with advanced lymphoedema (black arrow) with no drainage to the left axilla.

Near-infrared fluorescent lymphography (ICG lymphography)

Most centres do not routinely perform imaging on limbs with lymphoedema, but some of the larger or more research-focused lymphoedema centres may perform various specialised tests. For example, at the ALERT Centre, we perform **near-infrared fluorescent lymphography**, also called **indocyanine green (ICG) lymphography**.

This procedure involves injecting a tiny amount of ICG dye (also known as Verdye) just under the skin in the first and fifth web space at the base of your fingers and at the base of the palm where your hand joins your wrist. A near-infrared camera (Photodynamic Eye; Hamamatsu Photonics, Japan) is used to visualise the lymphatic pathways, without direct contact with the skin. The lymphatic vessels and fluid flow are illuminated, allowing us to mark the pathways directly onto the skin using a pen.

After marking the pathways, we apply gentle massage towards the armpit, encouraging the ICG dye to flow upwards through the arm, helping to map the direction of lymphatic fluid movement (**Figure 4.7**). The large green areas visible on the scan in stage 2 and 3 lymphoedema indicate dermal backflow – a sign of congestion where lymphatic fluid has built up and is attempting to bypass the disrupted lymphatic vessels.

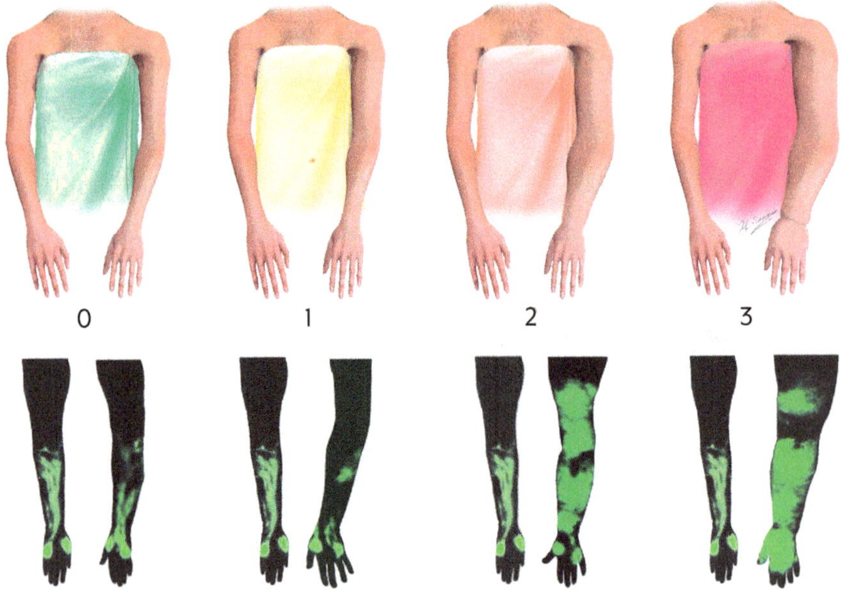

Figure 4.7

ICG lymphography scan of the left arm, by stage of lymphoedema. The large patches of green in stage 2 and 3 are showing "dermal backflow", where blocked circulation has caused congested lymphatic fluid to leak into the skin. Copyright Hiroo Suami, with permission.

In a publication for ALERT, world-leading expert in lymphatic anatomy A/Prof Hiroo Suami documented the lymphatic drainage of patients with breast or skin cancer, most of whom (93%) had been treated with an axillary dissection (Suami, 2018). Using advanced ICG imaging, he was able to identify the destination of the lymphatic fluid (drainage region) and specific routes taken by the fluid (drainage patterns).

These patterns were termed "original" or "compensatory". Original drainage patterns, as seen in the armpit and neck (**Figure 4.8**), show lymphatic fluid flowing in a normal direction before the onset of lymphoedema. Compensatory drainage patterns, as seen in the breastbone, opposite armpit and shoulder blade, signify abnormal lymphatic flow after the diagnosis of lymphoedema.

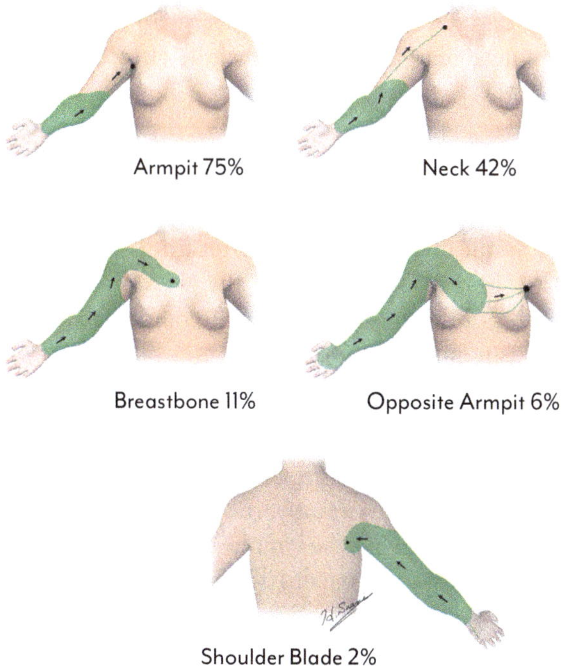

Figure 4.8

Pattern of lymphatic drainage for patients with lymphoedema after an axillary dissection, using indocyanine green (ICG) fluorescent lymphography: draining to the armpit (axilla), around the collarbone to the lower neck (clavicular), across the chest to the nodes behind the breastbone (internal mammary chain) or to the opposite axilla (Koelmeyer, 2021).

Over time, our team at ALERT built on this research to publish a larger analysis of ICG lymphography in 339 patients (Koelmeyer, 2021). For three out of four patients, lymphatic fluid still drained through the axilla, even though most axillary lymph nodes had been removed (**Figure 4.8**, top left). This confirmed that massage towards the armpit is still an important pathway for lymphatic drainage; the second most common drainage pattern used a "bypass pathway", following the outer edge of the arm to the lymph nodes at the neck (**Figure 4.8**, top right). Furthermore, no patients had drainage to groin lymph nodes, indicating that patients don't need **manual lymphatic drainage (MLD)** in that direction.

In the updated publication, we identified three main patterns of superficial compensation that allow for lymphatic drainage in and around congested areas, known as "dermal backflow bridging", "new vessel bridging" and "localised deep entry point". These patterns can often work together, enabling continued lymphatic drainage in limbs affected by lymphoedema (Koelmeyer, 2021).

For patients with resistant lymphoedema, ICG lymphography can help direct massage pathways and indicate the amount of pressure needed for lymphatic drainage. It can also help determine what sort of surgery is required, if applicable. Severe allergic reactions to ICG are rare, but the procedure is best avoided if you are allergic to shellfish or iodine. In Australia, the cost of this test is currently not reimbursed by Medicare or private health insurance.

I have been present for many ICG lymphography procedures. One of the main advantages is that you can see what is happening with the lymphatic circulation in your arm in real time, and how the fluid moves with gentle or firmer massage. Most importantly, the test identifies your individual lymphatic flow pattern, giving the lymphoedema therapist a roadmap to provide you with optimal, personalised care.

ALERT helped the lymphoedema team at the Princess Alexandria Hospital in Brisbane get its program off the ground, and I was pleased to see that they did some qualitative research into patients' reactions to this imaging test (Pigott, 2021). These reactions were overwhelmingly positive about the experience of ICG lymphography and its impact on their lymphoedema treatment: "It was just mind-blowing, to be honest" (Pigott, 2017).

Magnetic resonance imaging

Magnetic resonance imaging (MRI) has also been used for patients with lymphoedema, although it is not routinely done except at major lymphoedema centres.

In a study we conducted at the ALERT Centre, we used MRI to identify the amount of fat, lymphatic fluid and muscle in the arms of patients with arm lymphoedema, comparing their affected and unaffected sides (Sen and Boyages, 2018). As lymphoedema advances, more fat is deposited, and this can be easily seen on an MRI scan (Hoffner, 2018).

You may have had an MRI before, on other parts of your body. It is not an easy test, as the scanner can be noisy and feel a bit claustrophobic (**Figure 4.9** shows a picture of an MRI scanner). Patients are usually given earmuffs to suppress the noise.

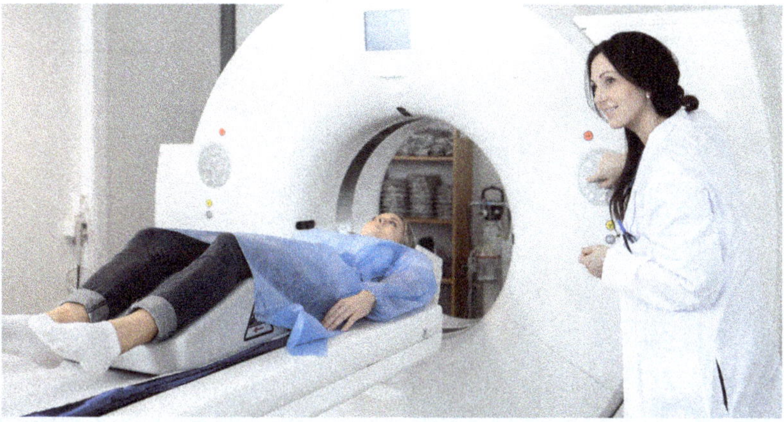

Figure 4.9
Magnetic resonance imaging (MRI) scanner.

Moisture meter

Many lymphoedema therapists use a specialised device called a **moisture meter** to measure the percentage water content under the skin. The LymphScanner (Delfin Technologies) is a hand-held device that uses a high-frequency electromagnetic wave to measure the "tissue dielectric constant", the ability of the tissue to store electrical energy (**Figure 4.10**). The display ranges from one to 80, with pure water having a value of 78.5. Measures are taken in multiple locations comparing the affected breast, arm, leg or other location to its unaffected counterpart.

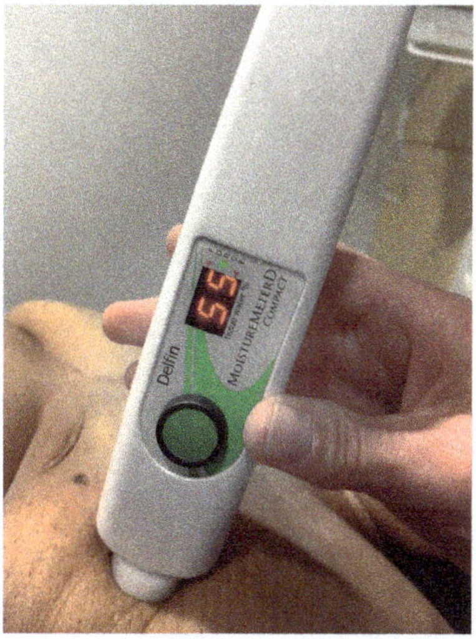

Figure 4.10
Moisture MeterD Compact (Delfin Technologies) showing increased water content in the lower part of the breast after breast conservation surgery.

Mapping the skin's water content with a moisture meter can be a quick way to identify the direction of lymphatic flow when ICG lymphography is not an option due to the time and expense involved (Czerniec, 2015).

5

EARLY DETECTION AND INTERVENTION

SHOULD I BE MONITORED FOR LYMPHOEDEMA?

The early warning signs of lymphoedema can be difficult to recognise, as some symptoms may overlap with temporary side effects from your initial surgery. Lymphoedema symptoms can also be vague and intermittent at first, or may be aggravated by heat, overuse or prolonged inactivity. You may notice some of the following symptoms in the affected limb, such as:

- A feeling of swelling or a change in the size of your arm, hand or breast
- Heaviness
- Aching, pain or tension
- Tightness or fullness
- Tightness of clothing, shoes or jewellery
- Transient swelling (swelling that comes and goes, and is more notice able at the end of the day)
- Numbness
- Skin changes.

Indents in the skin (pitting) caused by pressure from a bra, sleeve, garment or finger press (see **Figures 2.3** and **4.2**).

It is possible that your doctor may dismiss these signs or symptoms and advise you simply to learn to live with your new body. Take control and find an accredited **lymphoedema therapist** who can adequately assess and manage your symptoms. You may not have lymphoedema: aches and pains can occur from surgical scarring, or there may have been some nerve damage from your previous surgery. You may have cording (see **Figure 3.1**). However, it is important to get your symptoms checked out, as progressive lymphoedema can be irreversible.

CAN EARLY DETECTION AND TREATMENT HELP?

As with many medical conditions, including breast cancer, early detection and intervention can help to slow and potentially stop the progression of lymphoedema. Detection of subclinical lymphoedema can be picked up many months, even a year or two, before you or your doctor may have noticed a problem in your arm.

As mentioned earlier, I was fortunate to be one of the investigators in a large international multi-site clinical study with one of the world's foremost experts in lymphoedema, Professor Sheila Ridner. The PREVENT study evaluated 879 patients with breast cancer who were randomly allocated to close monitoring for lymphoedema, receiving regular arm measurements with either a tape measure or bioimpedance spectroscopy (Ridner, 2022).

The primary focus of PREVENT was on identifying subclinical lymphoedema: early, subtle signs of fluid build-up that appear before the lymphoedema becomes visible or symptomatic. If any such signs were detected, either by bioimpedance or tape measure, an intervention was initiated immediately. The intervention consisted of wearing a **ready-to-wear garment** for four weeks. This compression garment worked by applying graduated pressure to the affected area, helping the muscles to push excess lymphatic fluid away and preventing the fluid from accumulating further.

We found that there were more "false alarms" for lymphoedema in the tape measure group, causing unnecessary anxiety for those participants. Tape measurements can vary slightly between different practitioners, and arm size can change for reasons other than swelling, such as an increase in fat or muscle mass (see **Figure 4.4**). In this study, we found that our early intervention with four weeks of a graduated compression garment was often enough to actually reverse the subclinical lymphoedema.

Taking control means working with a good lymphoedema therapist who can monitor your limb using bioimpedance spectroscopy (if available), or using regular limb volume measurement with a tape measure or perometer (see **Figure 4.5**). You should see your lymphoedema therapist if you develop any symptoms in your affected limb that don't settle down. Ideally the therapist will be part of a multidisciplinary team, working closely with your surgeon and oncologists to provide pre- and postoperative care, as well as screening and early intervention for lymphoedema.

BIOIMPEDANCE SPECTROSCOPY AND L-DEX

Bioimpedance spectroscopy involves passing a harmless electric signal through your body to check the level of resistance in your tissue. Modern bioimpedance technology uses devices similar to a smart stand-up scale, which can measure the lymphatic fluid in your limb as well as your overall body composition. An example of this is the SOZO device, which has several

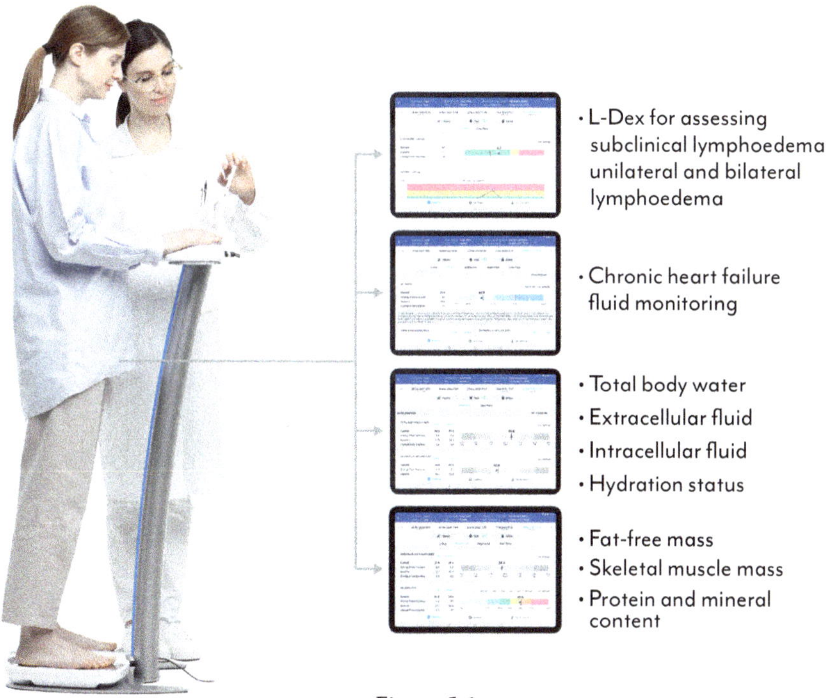
• L-Dex for assessing subclinical lymphoedema unilateral and bilateral lymphoedema
• Chronic heart failure fluid monitoring
• Total body water
• Extracellular fluid
• Intracellular fluid
• Hydration status
• Fat-free mass
• Skeletal muscle mass
• Protein and mineral content

Figure 5.1

The SOZO device is quick and convenient, and can measure body composition as well as lymphoedema.

available output types, including your protein content, hydration levels, muscle mass and fat-free mass (see **Figures 5.1–5.2**). Other instruments also exist that use bioimpedance to detect lymphoedema (Cho, 2020).

What does the L-Dex score mean?

L-Dex is a trademarked term for "lymphoedema index", and is a measurement of fluid build-up in a limb at risk of developing lymphoedema. The L-Dex score is a ratio of the resistance between your affected and unaffected limbs when the electric signal is passed through your body. The more fluid in your tissue spaces, the faster the current passes through them and the higher your L-Dex score.

Originally, clinical lymphoedema was defined as an L-Dex score of more than 10. The normal range is -10 to +10. In the PREVENT study, we used an increase in L-Dex score of greater than 6.5 units from the preoperative baseline to indicate subclinical lymphoedema. A person's baseline may

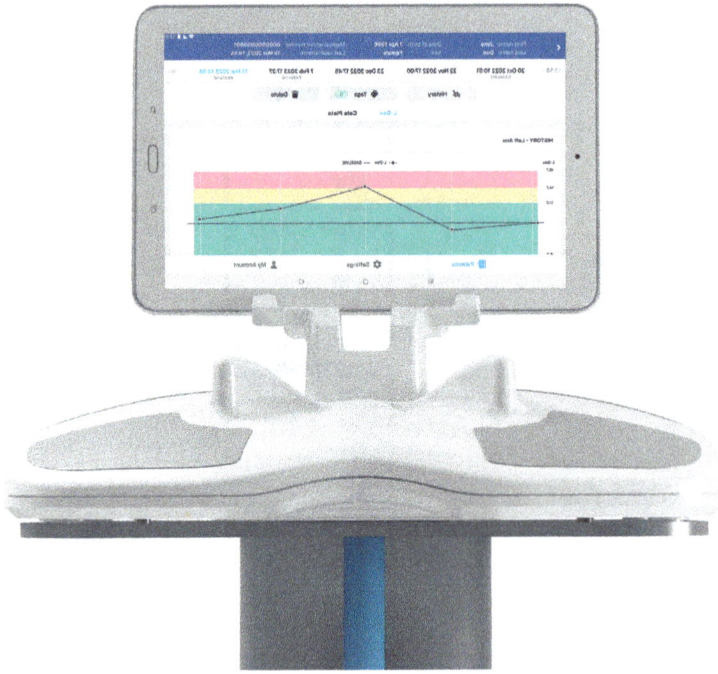

Figure 5.2

The SOZO device can graph multiple measurements of the L-Dex score.

even be a negative score; if your preoperative L-Dex is -2.0, we need to consider early intervention if it increases to +4.5 after surgery. If there is no preoperative baseline, subclinical lymphoedema is defined as a reading of around 7.0.

HOW FREQUENTLY SHOULD I BE MONITORED?

Well, it depends. First you need to be aware of your individual risk of lymphoedema, so that you can have screening more often if your risk is higher, and less often if it is lower. In Australia, we generally recommend a mammogram every two years for breast cancer screening, but would increase this to yearly if you had a strong family history or previous diagnosis of breast cancer. The same goes with lymphoedema screening – one size doesn't fit all. In the first year after surgery, it's a good idea to be monitored every three to six months so that early signs of lymphoedema can be detected before any symptoms occur.

In 2023, in collaboration with Professor Sheila Ridner from Vanderbilt University, Dr Frank Vicini from the University of Michigan, Dr Chirag Shah from the Cleveland Clinic, A/Prof Louise Koelmeyer and others, I wrote a paper about the risk factors for arm lymphoedema and how often patients should be monitored based on their individual risk (Boyages, 2023).

Here is a snapshot of our recommendations:

- Pre-treatment: A baseline measurement is advised, by L-Dex, tape-measure circumference or limb volume. I prefer the L-Dex score as a quick and easy method that works in my clinic, so I always use bioimpedance spectroscopy in my own work settings.
- Years 1–3: Three- to six-monthly screening, depending on the level of risk:
    - If low risk, such as a sentinel node biopsy (with only one or two nodes removed) and normal weight, six-monthly screening is probably enough.
    - If high risk, such as an ALND or radiation to the supraclavicular fossa, taxane chemotherapy or being obese or overweight, then three-monthly screening is ideal.
- Years 4–5: If you're considered low-risk and have no signs of lymphoedema, screening can stop, but you should keep an eye out for any symptoms such as heaviness, tingling, fullness, tight ness or pain in the limb.

Don't forget, it's important to make sure that your shoulder function also gets back to normal. This is expected within three months after your surgery. Information on shoulder care after breast cancer treatment can be found on the Westmead Breast Cancer Institute website: visit https://www.bci.org.au/breast-cancer-information/fact-sheets/shoulder-care/ (see also **Useful websites**, page 174).

6

COMPLEX LYMPHOEDEMA THERAPY

Complex lymphoedema therapy (CLT) is considered to be international best practice for managing lymphoedema (Haesler, 2016a). It may also be called **complete decongestive therapy** (CDT). The terms CLT and CDT are used interchangeably; in Australia, the primary term is CLT, which is what I've used in this book.

CLT is recommended as the first step in lymphoedema management, to rapidly reduce the swelling and decongest your affected limb (hence "decongestive therapy"). The primary goals of CLT are to reduce limb volume, prevent the progression of fibrosis and fat deposition, and maintain this reduction through ongoing self-management techniques. Another important goal is to improve quality of life by minimising the physical and psychological burden of lymphoedema. Effective CLT not only helps control the swelling in your arm or leg but also reduces your risk of developing complications such as cellulitis (see **Chapter 13**, Prevention and Treatment of Cellulitis). The goals of treatment need to be individualised for you. This will depend on multiple factors including your responsibilities at home or work, what you like to do, where you live and your level of support at home.

CLT has two phases: the reduction phase and the maintenance phase (**Table 6.1**). Many of the aspects are the same, with the maintenance phase being more self-directed rather than administered by a therapist.

COMPONENTS OF CLT	
Phase 1: Reduction	**Phase 2: Maintenance**
Assessment	Assessment
Education and support	Education and support
Skin care	Skin care
Manual lymphatic drainage (MLD)	Self MLD +/ periodic therapist MLD
Compression (bandaging, garments)	Compression (garments +/ sequential intermittent compression pumps)
Exercise	Exercise

Table 6.1

Components of treatment with complex lymphoedema therapy (CLT).

PHASE 1: REDUCTION PHASE

Phase 1, the reduction phase, involves intensive treatment by a lymphoedema therapist to decongest your limb. It is also known as the intensive phase. As shown in **Table 6.1**, phase 1 involves skin care with a good moisturiser, manual lymphatic drainage (a form of massage to improve lymphatic flow, referred to as MLD), compression therapy (with bandaging or a reduction compression garment), exercise to boost circulation and, of course, education and psychosocial support. For subclinical or mild cases of lymphoedema, it's possible that treatment may only consist of a compression garment with or without MLD, omitting the reduction phase.

The way the reduction phase is done varies by country, by therapist, and most importantly by patient, according to your individual needs. A/Prof Koelmeyer from the ALERT Centre states that "international best practice is four to six weeks of daily MLD, intensive bandaging, skin care, exercise and psychological support". While CLT with daily bandaging is considered the gold standard, this may not always be possible for your situation. Modified CLT may involve a week or two in hospital or at a rehabilitation centre, or daily visits to a lymphoedema therapist for more established lymphoedema symptoms. A combination of treatment modalities is also possible in this phase. For example, your lymphoedema therapist may apply compression bandages two to three times a week, and you can use a compression pump or even self-bandage over a garment between therapist treatments.

Assessment

The most important part of lymphoedema management is the initial assessment. This is why a new consultation is usually longer and more expensive than a follow-up consultation. Your lymphoedema therapist will want to know all about your personal situation, including your medical and family history; your cancer treatment and lymph node involvement; how long you've had lymphoedema and how it's affecting you, and whether you have had any episodes of cellulitis. Assessment also includes a physical examination and various measurements described in **Chapter 4**, Clinical Assessment and Tests. The therapist will also prioritise your personal treatment goals.

Treatment by a lymphoedema therapist is designed to help you achieve the following outcomes:

- Prevent progression of your lymphoedema
- Reduce swelling in the limb, and maintain the reduction
- Reduce your risk of infection (usually cellulitis, but also fungal skin infections)
- Improve your limb function and quality of life
- Reduce thickening of the skin (fibrosis)
- Empower you to feel in control and potentially manage your lymphoedema independently.

Education and support

In addition to the physical components of CLT, you should receive specialist advice, education and psychosocial support. This may include information on skin care, exercise, nutrition and other lifestyle factors that can impact lymphoedema. You may also receive psychological support to help you cope with the challenges of living with lymphoedema.

It's mentally tough to make it through cancer treatment only to end up with lymphoedema, and having periods of feeling down is normal (see **Chapter 15**, The Emotional Side of Lymphoedema). Let your care team know how you are feeling, as there are many ways that they can help. Understanding your condition is part of the solution, and it is vital that you see an accredited lymphoedema therapist to guide you through this phase of your care. It's important to have the support of people close to you, such as family or friends.

I have seen many of my patients successfully learn to adapt to the changes in their body caused by lymphoedema. On the other hand, many patients are devastated by a lymphoedema diagnosis and seek as much information and treatment as possible. It is important not to rush into treatments that seem too good to be true. Taking control means understanding your condition and adopting a trial-and-error approach under qualified supervision. You may like to visit some of the websites listed at the end of this book for more information (see page 174).

Education includes understanding that lymphoedema is not curable. Having lymphoedema is a bit like having diabetes – you can control it, but you can't cure it, especially if it's not treated early. It's important to take care of your body to help manage your lymphoedema. Try and keep your weight under control and restrict your consumption of sugary fluids and processed foods; build up your muscle strength and look after your skin. Record your arm volume or L-Dex measurements in the same way that someone with diabetes would monitor their blood glucose level.

Skin care

Skin care is a crucial component of CLT, as lymphoedema increases the risk of infection and other skin-related issues. Healthy, intact skin protects against infection. Keep your skin clean and moisturised, avoid harsh soaps or perfumes and protect your skin from cuts, scratches, insect bites and sunburn. Inspect your skin regularly so you can be alert to any signs of infection, such as redness, warmth or swelling, and seek medical attention promptly if these symptoms occur. I will discuss skin care more (as well as nail care) in **Chapter** 7, Skin Care and Lymphoedema.

Manual lymphatic drainage

Manual lymphatic drainage (MLD) encourages congested fluid to move from the part of the body with "blocked" or non-functional lymphatic vessels towards functional lymphatic vessels. The lymphatic fluid then makes its way to the thoracic duct in the centre of your body, and from there, it can drain back into the large veins at the base of your neck (see **Figure 1.1** for an overview of the lymphatic system). MLD is often used as an important step before compression. There are various techniques for MLD that are taught across the world; since the knowledge of lymphatic anatomy is important for successful MLD, it should be performed by an accredited lymphoedema therapist (**Figure 6.1**). You may be able to do it yourself at home once your therapist has taught you the techniques.

MLD follows the pathways of the lymphatic system, including original and compensatory patterns, to help move lymphatic fluid towards lymph nodes that have not been affected by cancer treatment. ICG lymphography can detect abnormal pathways in affected areas (see **Figure 4.8**), allowing lymphoedema therapists to develop personalised massage routines and prescribe appropriate compression garments.

The therapist starts by using pressure to stimulate functioning lymph nodes in the drainage region for that body part, before focusing on the affected area. Incorporating deep breathing helps by enhancing the movement of your diaphragm and facilitating the flow of lymphatic fluid in the abdominal region (Iannello, 2020). There are various types of massage strokes. Usually, the pressure is slow and firm over areas of dermal backflow or congestion, with short strokes moving towards the drainage region (for example, from arm to axilla or leg to groin). Elevation is also helpful and can be used to facilitate drainage.

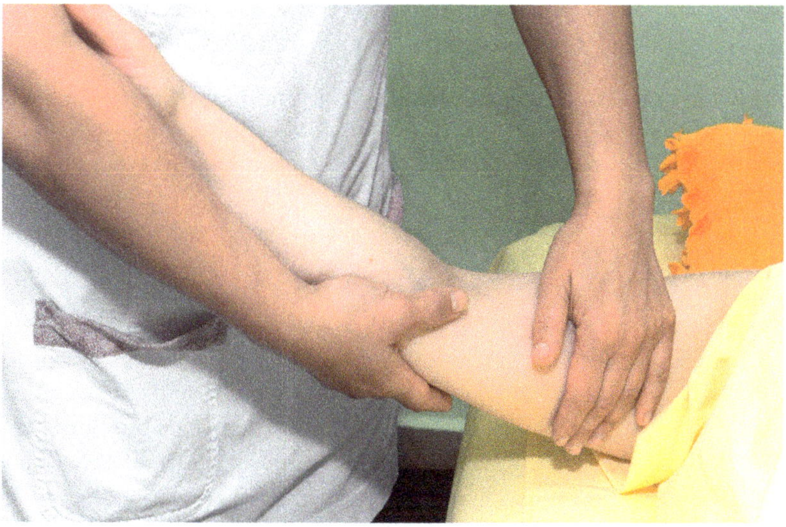

Figure 6.1

Phase 1 of CLT involves manual lymphatic drainage to decongest the arm.

While MLD has been widely practised for lymphoedema management, recent evidence calls its effectiveness into question. Some research, including studies by De Vrieze (2022) and Devoogdt (2023), suggests that MLD may have limited impact on reducing arm volume and improving skin elasticity or fibrosis in breast cancer-related lymphoedema. These findings indicate that we should focus instead on multi-layer lymphoedema bandaging and the use of tailored compression garments, which have been found to be more effective. In some countries, practitioners have adopted this compression-focused approach instead of MLD. Professor Brorson states: "In Sweden, no MLD is given in hospitals. The focus is on bandaging and compression, and therefore therapists can treat more patients when omitting MLD."

In Australia, the US and elsewhere, MLD remains a standard practice. At ALERT, we use a more targeted method of MLD by incorporating ICG lymphography. Once the ICG has provided a road map of where the lymphatic fluid is draining and how it travels (the drainage region and pattern), we can determine the most appropriate use of MLD, including the ideal amount of pressure and whether it should be self-directed or therapist-guided. A/Prof Koelmeyer notes that "more research is required into the effectiveness of MLD. Historically, a gentle massage technique was taught, but now with ICG we see that massage needs to be firmer in areas of congestion and dermal backflow" (Koelmeyer, 2021).

MLD has been associated with reduced pain and improved function and quality of life (Haesler, 2016a). However, while it's one of the approaches in our lymphoedema toolkit, the most important component is undoubtably compression (Haesler, 2016b).

Compression

Compression is the single most important element of lymphoedema care. The aim is to reduce the swelling in your arm or other affected area until it's as close to normal as possible. Water moves because of the force applied to it. Toothpaste comes out of a tube when squeezed, and your lymphatic vessels work in a similar way. Compression therapy works with the shape of your limb and the muscles underneath to create a pressure gradient that helps shift accumulated lymphatic fluid out of the swollen and congested body part. Every time your muscles contract, they push fluid through and around the disrupted lymphatic vessels, similar to squeezing a sponge.

Compression can be applied in a variety of ways: the most common methods are bandaging or wearing a compression garment. Compression devices such as **sequential intermittent pneumatic compression** (SIPC) pumps are used in the maintenance phase of CLT, which will be covered in the next section. The goal of compression in the reduction phase is to achieve maximum reduction in limb volume, promoting lymphatic circulation to reduce swelling and ensure comfort during your daily activities. The main method used in the reduction phase is compression bandaging.

In the reduction phase of CLT, short-stretch compression bandages play a vital role. During this phase, the shape and size of the limb change daily, so external compression needs to be adjustable. Made from low-elasticity materials, short-stretch bandages provide safe, adjustable and fully customisable compression to the affected area. They apply lower pressure when the limb is at rest, but increase pressure significantly with movement, creating dynamic compression that works with muscle activity to promote lymphatic drainage and reduce swelling.

Multi-layer lymphoedema bandaging (**Figure 6.2**) allows for daily treatment as part of the reduction phase. This bandaging system typically consists of an inner comfort layer that provides padding and absorbs moisture, and an outer compression layer that delivers controlled pressure to reduce swelling. To begin, a tubular gauze is applied over moisturised skin to protect it from direct contact with the layers above. This is followed by a layer of soft padding or foam to cushion any bony areas, distribute pressure evenly and prevent a tourniquet effect, ensuring safe and effective compression. The short-stretch bandage is then applied over the top as the outer layer. The different materials work together, with the comfort layer providing support and the short-stretch compression layer creating the necessary pressure for managing the swelling.

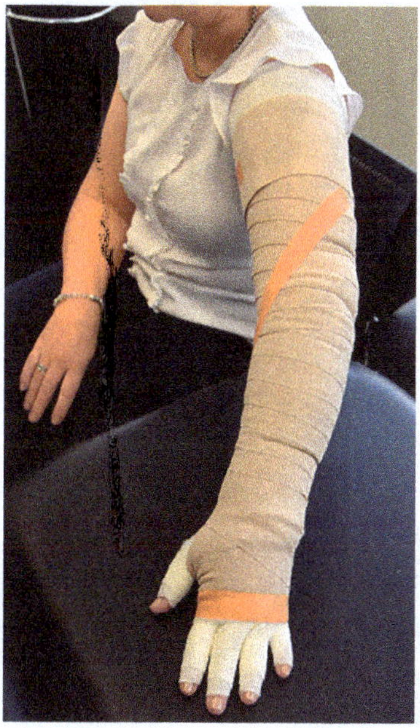

Figure 6.2

Compression in phase 1 of CLT (reduction phase) using a multi-layer short-stretch bandage application. This is done every day for two weeks as an inpatient or outpatient.

Most patients prefer to undergo bandaging as an outpatient during their intensive reduction phase. Two-layer short-stretch bandage application allows for treatment two to three times per week, making it ideal for those who find it challenging to attend daily sessions and prefer not to be admitted as an inpatient (Moffatt, 2012). This two-layer bandage technology is offered by all the major brands, including the 3M Coban range, Jobst Compri2 and others. These types of companies offer specialised products and have advisors to help you choose the right system and learn proper application techniques, in conjunction with your lymphoedema therapist. In two-layer short-stretch bandaging for arm lymphoedema, the process begins by bandaging the fingers and hand (**Figure 6.3**), followed by the entire arm (**Figure 6.4**).

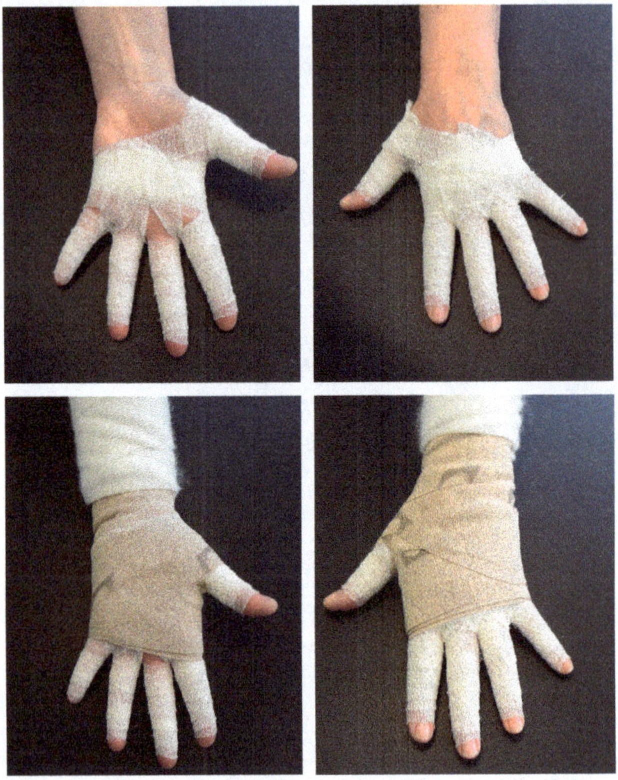

Figure 6.3

Compression in phase 1 of CLT using a two-layer short-stretch bandage application, starting with the hand. This type of bandaging is done two to three times a week.

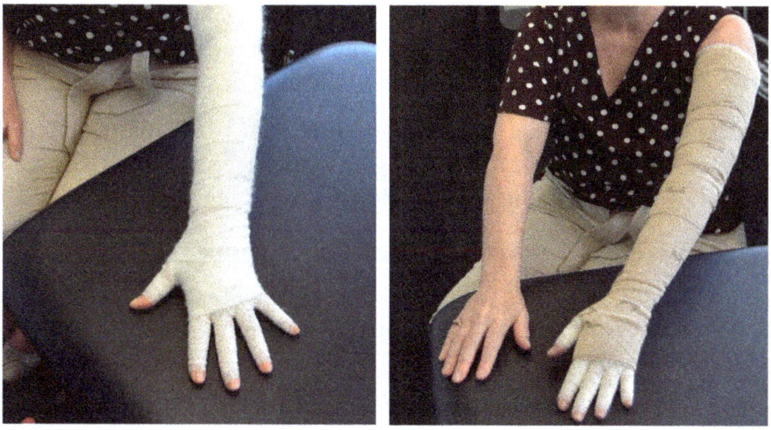

Figure 6.4

Two-layer short-stretch bandage application extending from the hand to the axilla (armpit).

Alternatively, a Velcro adjustable compression garment using short overlapping strips may be easier to manage at home, if you can't tolerate bandaging and you have someone to help you apply the wrap. Examples include, in alphabetical order, the Haddenham easywrap, Jobst FarrowWrap, Juzo Compression Wrap and Medi Circaid Wrap. These wraps can be fiddly to use but work well for patients with significant shoulder immobility (e.g. due to arthritis), and are commonly used for swollen legs. An example of a wrap garment system is shown in **Figure 6.5** below. When using an arm wrap compression system, it is vital that a hand wrap is also used to prevent fluid building up in the hand.

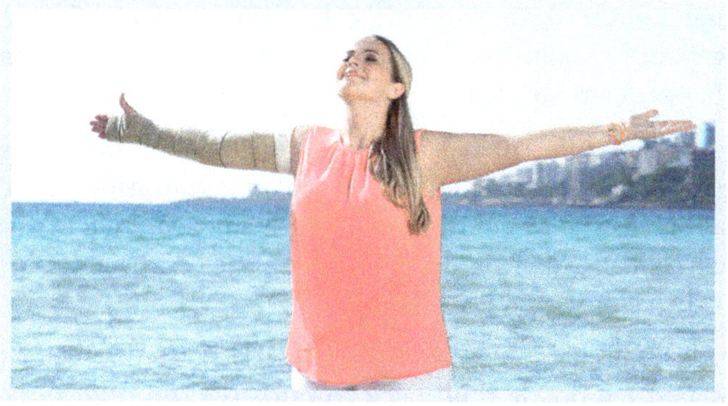

Figure 6.5

Example of an arm wrap compression system (Circaid Juxtafit system).
Copyright Medi Australia, with permission.

Remember, these bandages are not waterproof, so take care to keep them dry. If you experience any pain or numbness, let your therapist know right away, as this could indicate improper application or excessive pressure.

Having a fully wrapped or bandaged limb can make many activities awkward, and you may find it challenging to manage your usual daily tasks. The following tips may help you during the reduction phase of your CLT:

- Stock up on groceries ahead of time to ensure you have what you need at home.
- Make sure your laundry is up to date before starting treatment.
- Prepare a few meals in advance and store them in the freezer for easy access.
- To avoid getting your bandages wet, consider sponge baths during the intensive phase, or plan your showers right before your therapy appointments.
- If your arm is bandaged, try wearing a shoulder-length examination glove or garbage bag over your arm in the shower to keep it dry.
- If your leg is bandaged, buy adjustable sandals or footwear that can accommodate the extra bulk, as your regular shoes may not fit.
- Bandages can be bulky, so wear loose-fitting clothing to your appointments to make dressing easier.

Exercise

In general, exercise encourages muscle movement, which in turn helps to boost your lymphatic circulation. Get to know your new body and determine what amount of exercise works for you.

There are many different types of exercise: aerobic (cardio), resistance (strength), flexibility (stretching) and balance (proprioception). Each has its advantages; for example, stretching is a type of exercise that won't increase lymphatic fluid production. Exercise is beneficial for managing lymphoedema for several reasons:

When your muscles contract, they create resistance that helps to push accumulated lymphatic fluid back towards the centre of the body to promote drainage. Wearing a compression garment while exercising increases this resistance.

Deep breathing during exercise moves your diaphragm up and down, pushing fluid towards the large lymphatic vessels where it drains back into the bloodstream. This movement of the diaphragm is a bit like using a plunger to unblock a clogged drain.

Moving and stretching your body activates the lymphatic capillaries and promotes contraction of the lymphangions – small units or segments inside the capillaries – to improve the lymphatic circulation. (See **Chapter 1**, Understanding the Lymphatic System, for more about lymphatic vessels and circulation.)

The most sensible approach is a slow, gradual progression of exercise. Our bones, tendons and ligaments get stronger when stress is applied, and become weaker in the absence of stress. It's also important to cool down by doing some gentle exercise with the same muscles you just used during your work-out: for example, if you run for 30 minutes, follow this with another 10–15 minutes of slow walking to cool down.

If you have lymphoedema, compression should be worn during exercise if tolerated – keeping your garment on gives your muscles extra support as they push the lymphatic fluid along your limb. If you're uncomfortable exercising with your garment on, try putting it on right after you've finished exercising. Some of my patients wear black-coloured compression garments when they exercise, as it is less obvious and feels more "sporty".

In 2018, the Clinical Oncology Society of Australia (COSA) published comprehensive exercise guidelines for cancer patients, recommending at least 150 minutes of moderate-intensity aerobic exercise (such as brisk walking, jogging, swimming or cycling) per week, and two to three sessions of strength training per week with exercises targeting major muscle groups (Cormie, 2018). Some healthcare professionals voiced concerns that their patients could not achieve this level of exercise (Newton, 2018), which led COSA to soften their stance a bit in later updates. Just do the best you can, and seek help from a personal trainer or exercise physiologist if you can afford the extra expense. You can access COSA's exercise guidelines on their website: visit https://www.cosa.org.au/advocacy/position-statements/exercise-in-cancer-care/ (see also **Useful websites**, page 174).

More information about exercise is discussed in **Chapter 12**, Lymphoedema Precautions – Fact vs Fiction.

PHASE 2: MAINTENANCE PHASE

Phase 2 starts immediately after phase 1 and aims to maintain the results achieved by your intensive treatment.

Table 6.1 shows that both phases are essentially the same, but phase 2 requires more involvement from you and less from your therapist. In the maintenance phase, lymphoedema becomes largely self-managed, with periodic assessments and MLD performed by an accredited lymphoedema therapist.

The most important element of self-care in this phase is wearing a compression garment that has been prescribed, measured and fitted by a qualified lymphoedema therapist. Other strategies include skin care, infection prevention, self-massage and exercise (see **Table 6.1**). Many patients also add sequential intermittent pneumatic compression (SIPC) to their treatment regimen, which is compression using a lymphoedema massage pump. You can use the pump for an hour once or twice a day while sitting in a comfortable chair. This time can vary; A/Prof Louise Koelmeyer notes that most of her patients use the pump once a day for 45 minutes. You can discuss the optimal time with your therapist and come up with a routine that works for you.

Managing swelling during the maintenance phase can be supported by night-time compression garments with textured surfaces, which provide gentle, gradient compression while resting (**Figure 6.6** and **10.3**). Examples include, in alphabetical order, the Haddenham Comfiwave, Jobst Relax, Juzo SoftCompress, Medi Circaid Juxtafit Essentials and Circaid Profile, and Solaris TributeNight.

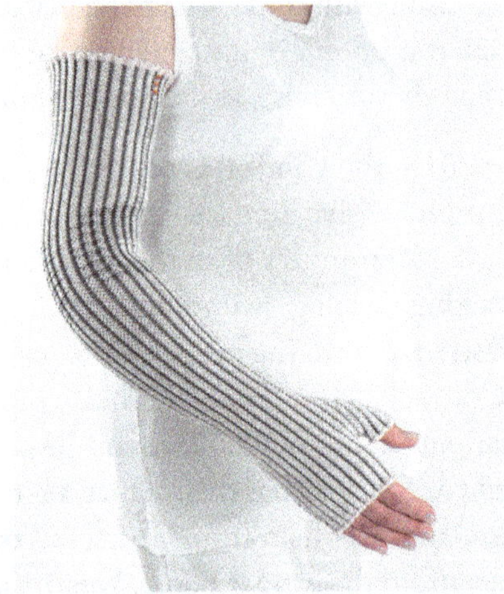

Figure 6.6

Example of a night-time compression garment: the Haddenham Comfiwave. Copyright Haddenham Healthcare Limited, 2025, with permission.

These garments, often made from soft, breathable materials, are more comfortable than traditional bandaging and not as restrictive as daytime garments. They are generally easy to put on and take off. Less bulky than other options, they allow for better mobility and, if needed, can be worn under regular clothing. When combined with an SIPC pump (discussed below), night-time garments form an important part of the maintenance phase of lymphoedema management. However, specialised night-time garments can be more costly than traditional bandages.

Sequential intermittent pneumatic compression

Sequential intermittent pneumatic compression (SIPC) pumps have been used for many years to treat lymphoedema. They are designed to improve lymphatic flow and reduce swelling by applying rhythmic pressure to the affected area. An SIPC pump consists of an inflatable sleeve placed around the affected area and attached to a machine which inflates and deflates it in a sequence (hence the term "sequential"). For arm lymphoedema, the sequence usually starts at your hand, with the pumping action moving in an upwards direction towards the armpit (**Figure 6.7**). SIPC pumps can also be used on the chest wall or breast (**Figure 6.8**), trunk, arms or legs.

SIPC is a great tool to help flush sluggish or slow-flowing lymphatic fluid out of your limb or chest area. There have been significant improvements in the design and technology of SIPC pumps for lymphoedema over the last ten years. The pumps are portable and easy to use; many patients report that they enjoy the convenience of a home pump and find it relaxing to use. For added benefit, you can wear a textured night-time compression garment at the time of pumping.

You should not use a pump without guidance from a lymphoedema therapist. Don't just buy one off the internet and start using it without instruction or supervision. You need to make sure that you're using it correctly, so that the pump doesn't lead to fluid accumulating and the tissue thickening at the top of your arm. If your lymphoedema therapist recommends SIPC as part of your treatment plan, they will trial a pump with you as the first step. After that, it is a good idea to rent one first so you can try it out at home. If you find that the pump is helpful, you may consider a longer-term rental or purchase, depending on your financial situation.

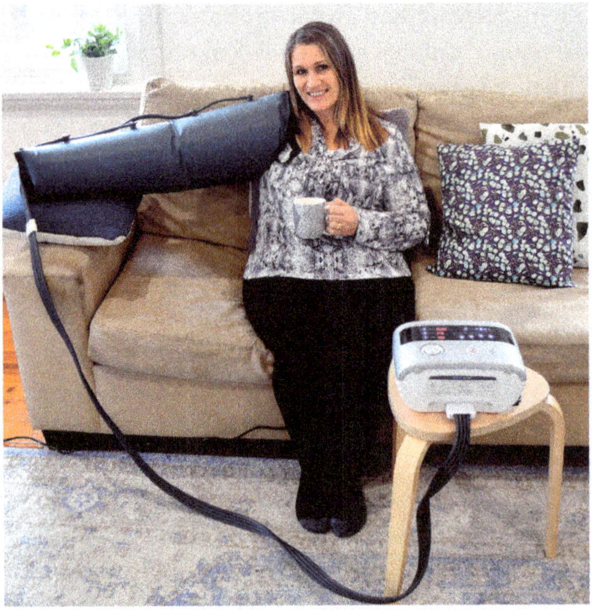

Figure 6.7

Phase 2 of CLT involving a home-based sequential intermittent pneumatic compression (SIPC) arm pump. Copyright Medi Rent Australia, with permission.

Several small studies have compared SIPC to manual lymphatic drainage (MLD) and found that the two approaches have similar benefits for lymphoedema (Uzkeser, 2015). One clinical trial in Turkey compared 24 patients treated with a compression garment and MLD to 22 patients treated with a compression garment and SIPC pump (Sanal-Toprak, 2019). The patients had their respective treatment for five weeks, then after the fifth week they continued with just the garment and a home exercise program. The results showed no significant difference between the two groups: all patients had significant improvement in their arm circumference and shoulder mobility, as well as improved symptoms of pain, tightness and heaviness. In other words, MLD and SIPC were found to be equally effective as components of CLT. These treatments can be used on the arm, leg or breast, as well as in the head and neck region (Ridner, 2021).

One of the main advantages of SIPC that my patients tell me is that it allows them to take control – by using a pump at home, they can do their lymphatic drainage in their own time, rather than needing to attend a therapist, often during work hours, for frequent sessions of MLD. Professor Sheila Ridner adds that "SIPC makes lymphoedema therapy more accessible to those in rural areas who cannot come into larger population areas frequently to get CLT". The key point, however, is that SIPC cannot be effective on its own; it must be used with a properly fitted and functioning compression garment. An old or worn-out garment that no longer provides adequate pressure won't deliver the intended benefits. It's essential to have a garment that maintains the necessary compression levels for effective lymphoedema management.

Managing compression garments

It's important that you can self-manage in the maintenance phase, as you will not have as much close involvement from your therapist. There are various products available to make it easier to wear your garment consistently. Silicone bands or strips can be a great addition, as they prevent the garment from slipping or rolling by providing a secure grip against your skin. If you need extra hold, applying skin glue can also improve adherence and keep your garment in place throughout the day, especially on parts of the body that move frequently. Shoulder straps are another option to consider – they provide extra support to keep your garment from slipping, which can be particularly helpful for arm lymphoedema. Finally, think about whether you can get assistance from family members or community carers, as managing compression garments typically requires support twice a day, every day. This can sometimes be difficult to organise, but it can make a big difference in keeping up with your treatment.

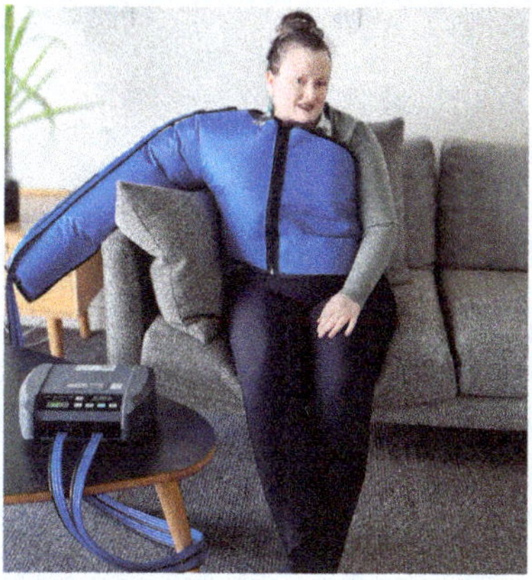

Figure 6.8

Phase 2 of CLT involving a home-based SIPC arm and vest pump. Copyright Medi Rent Australia, with permission.

7

SKIN CARE AND LYMPHOEDEMA

Skin care is an essential part of complex lymphoedema therapy (CLT), as lymphoedema can cause changes to the skin, making it more prone to infection. The skin can become dry, scaly and thickened. Keeping your skin clean and well-moisturised is vital to prevent dryness, cracking and other problems that can lead to infection.

Common clinical signs often seen in lymphoedema include skin changes such as thickening of the skin (hyperkeratosis), the development of small, wart-like growths (papillomatosis), rough or leathery skin (dermal lichenification), redness and swelling (**lymphoedema rubra**), and fluid leaking from the skin (**lymphorrhoea**). In more severe cases of lymphoedema, the skin may become hard and bumpy. Other skin-related issues that commonly present in lymphoedema include inflammation of hair follicles (folliculitis), infection of the lymphatic vessels (**lymphangitis**), bacterial skin infection (cellulitis), and long-lasting patches of thickened skin due to scratching (lichen simplex chronicum) (Fife, 2017).

Skin care is an integral part of CLT, and should include daily cleansing with gentle, pH-balanced soap and lukewarm water. Harsh soaps and hot water can damage your skin and lead to further complications. A bath or shower that leaves your skin pink is too hot and may exacerbate your lymphoedema. Keep baths or showers short. If you prefer to bathe, use a bath oil that is gentle on the skin; however, be very careful when stepping out of the bath, as oils can make surfaces slippery. Examples of suitable bath oils include QV Bath Oil, Aveeno Skin Relief Shower and Bath Oil, MooGoo Milk Wash, and Alpha Keri Shower and Bath Oil.

Pat your skin dry gently with a soft towel to avoid rubbing or friction. Moisturise your skin regularly with a gentle, fragrance-free lotion to help maintain its elasticity and reduce the risk of cracking.

It is also important to protect your skin from sunburn, cuts, scratches and other injuries that can exacerbate lymphoedema or increase your risk of infection. Insect bites can lead to skin infections, so wear protective clothing such as gloves and long sleeves or pants while gardening or when outside during the summer months, and use insect repellent. Wear oven mitts and long sleeves to protect your skin while using the oven. I will discuss this further in **Chapter 12**, Lymphoedema Precautions – Fact vs Fiction.

Avoid using razors where you've had extensive lymph node surgery, as loss of sensation in the area can make it hard to recognise small cuts which may introduce infection. Use an electric shaver instead in those areas. Waxing, depilatory creams or laser hair removal are reasonable alternatives, but keep a close eye on your skin for any signs of developing infection (see **Chapter 13**, Prevention and Treatment of Cellulitis).

WHY IS HYDRATING MY SKIN IMPORTANT?

Lymphoedema dries out the skin. Moisturisers can act as a shield to hydrate your skin and keep it healthy. They help your skin feel soft and smooth, and they are especially important if your skin becomes thickened by lymphoedema, because they can reduce the dryness and discomfort that often comes with swelling.

Terence Ryan, Emeritus Professor of Dermatology from Oxford University, has studied skin care in swollen limbs in several different countries (Ryan, 2013, 2017). He notes that when the epidermis (your skin's surface) is healthy, it provides excellent protection, helps to control body temperature and doesn't cause discomfort.

The outermost layer of the epidermis is called the **stratum corneum** and is often referred to as the skin's "barrier". It is composed of a tough, protective shield of dead skin cells. Bacteria and other debris that accumulate on the surface of your skin are removed as your body sheds and replaces the dead skin cells. The stratum corneum acts as a defence against external elements, such as harmful microorganisms and chemicals. It also retains moisture in your skin, preventing it from drying out.

It is essential to your skin's natural protection to keep the stratum corneum healthy and functioning. However, when it becomes unhealthy as a result of lymphoedema, the stratum corneum looks different and doesn't work properly. It triggers a repair process in the immune system that requires a lot of oxygen and releases substances called cytokines. The cytokines cause inflammation, which affects the deeper layers of the skin and brings more white blood cells to the area. So taking good care of your skin when you have lymphoedema is vital for your overall health and comfort.

It is important to moisturise your skin daily, using gentle pressure. Lymphatic capillaries do not have pumps and valves that contract like some of the larger lymphatic vessels, so you need to use gentle massage and exercise to manually assist the movement and drainage of fluid towards the lymph nodes. For example, if you have lymphoedema in your arm, apply the moisturiser using sweeping strokes towards your armpit. Your lymphoedema therapist can show you some techniques for moving the lymphatic fluid towards your axilla.

WHAT MOISTURISERS SHOULD I USE?

There are many different moisturisers available. If you're not sure which one to buy, talk to your local pharmacist. However, one factor to consider is the pH value of the product. According to Professor Ryan, "It should be remembered that the skin prefers to be acidic and that many soaps are very alkaline" (Ryan, 2017). This is why some people develop "dishwasher hands", where their skin reacts to the alkaline nature of dishwashing liquids and becomes irritated.

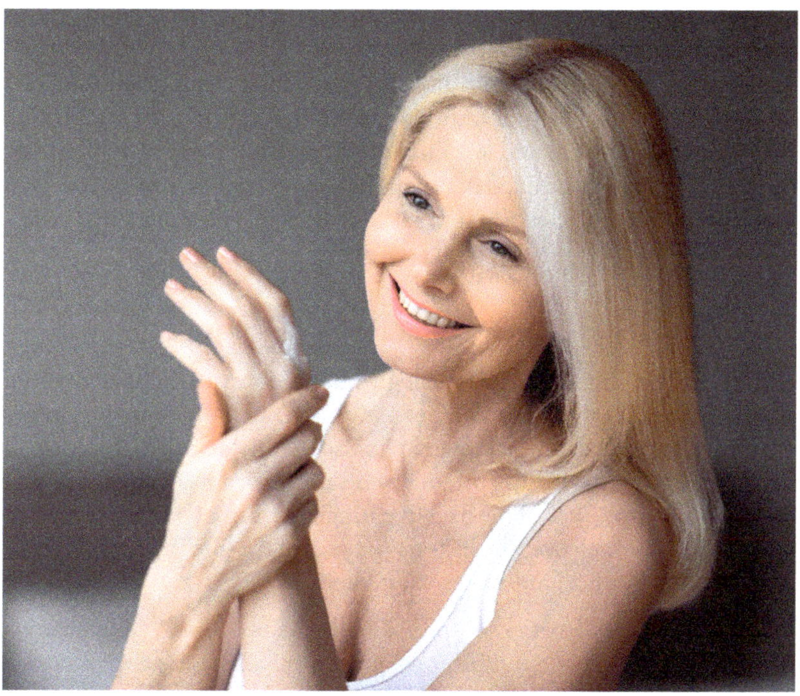

Figure 7.1

Ask your qualified therapist about how to moisturise your body area affected by lymphoedema.

The pH value of a substance indicates whether it is acidic or alkaline: a pH value of less than seven means the substance is acidic, and greater than seven means it is alkaline. Skin tends to be slightly acidic, with a pH of approximately four to six, while the inside of our bodies is close to neutral (pH 7). There is, therefore, a noticeable difference in pH between the surface of the skin and the layers underneath.

We now know that skin pH affects the essential enzymes that maintain healthy skin, so we're starting to understand that pH is critical to the way our skin functions and stays healthy (Ali, 2013). This study by Ali measured the pH levels of various moisturisers, including Cetaphil (pH 4.7), Aveeno (pH 5.6), Eucerin (pH 5.4) and Dove (pH 6.5), which were all in the acidic range. Check the fine print of your moisturiser to ensure it is also in the acidic range, preferably pH 4–6.

Coconut oil is a natural option that many people with lymphoedema find beneficial for their skin. Professor Ridner notes that "Coconut oil is cheap, has anti-inflammatory and antibacterial properties, smells good, and is used, based on anecdotal reports, with success by many lymphedoema patients. It is also natural with no additives". Pure coconut oil used as a moisturiser may be a helpful addition to your skin care routine, supporting the health of your skin and keeping it hydrated and protected. However, be sure to let the oil completely soak in before you put on your garment; if coconut oil gets onto compression garments it can affect their effectiveness and durability (Deen, 2021).

SHOULD I USE ANTIBACTERIAL CREAMS?

If you have lymphoedema, it is generally not necessary to use **antibacterial** skin products. However, if you get a cut or scratch on your skin in the affected area, an antibacterial cream or lotion may help prevent infection. If I get a scratch on my hand, I often rub the area with a good hand sanitiser, which can destroy 99% of the bacteria, fungi and viruses on our skin. Keep an eye on the scratch over the next few days to make sure it doesn't become hot, red or painful, all indicators of an infection.

Your lymphoedema therapist is probably the best person to advise you on the right products for your skin. Some practitioners advise against products that are too oily, as the oils can damage your compression garments, so use lotions rather than creams if possible. In **Chapter 13**, Prevention and Treatment of Cellulitis, I will discuss some of the research on using skin disinfectants.

WHEN SHOULD I USE ANTIFUNGAL PRODUCTS?

You may need to use an **antifungal** cream, lotion or powder if you develop a fungal skin infection in a part of the body where you have lymphoedema. Fungal infections can cause itching, redness and scaliness. Fungal infections of the skin (**Figure 7.2A**) are sometimes called "tinea" and can also involve the nail (**Figure 7.2B**). It's important to treat fungal infections, as they can compromise your skin integrity and create a pathway for bacterial infection. Fungal infections are extremely contagious and may spread to other areas of the skin, so you will need to use careful hygiene practices such as washing and thoroughly drying the area, not sharing towels, and washing clothes that are in contact with the affected area after each wear.

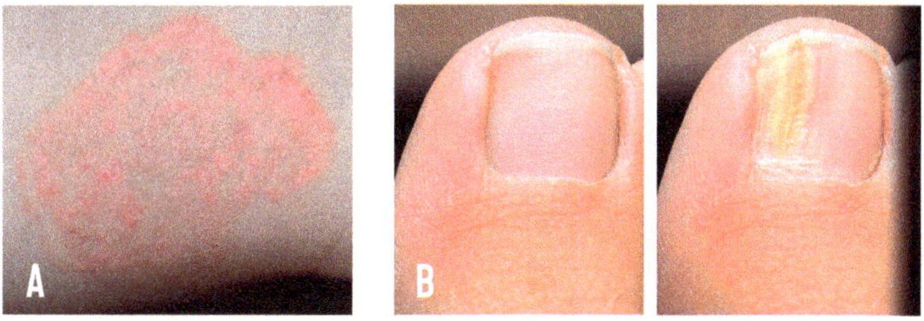

Figure 7.2

Typical tinea fungal rash of the skin (A) and fungal infection of a nail before and after treatment (B).

You must talk to your doctor or pharmacist before using antifungal products to ensure that they are appropriate for you. Sometimes antifungal tablets are required, if topical product like creams are not working. You may need referral to a dermatologist (skin specialist) if your rash is not responding to treatment, and the dermatologist may take a small biopsy or a scraping to be sent for analysis.

8

ALL ABOUT COMPRESSION GARMENTS

Choosing the right compression garment is not easy. It is best done in consultation with an accredited lymphoedema therapist, rather than simply buying one online. Compression garments used for lymphoedema are different from the "support stockings" or "anti-embolism stockings" sold in pharmacies, as these don't provide enough pressure to effectively manage lymphoedema.

Factors to consider include your age, activity level, occupation, body type, weight and skin condition; the severity of your lymphoedema, the shape of your limb, your tolerance to external compression and your ability to "**don**" (put on) and "**doff**" (take off) your garment. Lymphoedema therapists take this all into account when prescribing a compression garment.

You should also consider how much support you have at home. If you are older or somewhat frail, or if you suffer from arthritis or pain in your joints, it can be tricky to get a compression garment on and off without help. If your limb is large or distorted in shape, it can be difficult to get an adequate level of compression. Cost is another consideration, as compression garments can be expensive, and you need to replace them regularly.

The use of compression garments is the most practical and commonly used form of compression therapy. Other forms of compression therapy, such as bandaging or sequential intermittent pneumatic compression (SIPC), may be used during intensive stages of management to reduce swelling. For more about these techniques, see **Chapter 6**, Complex Lymphoedema Therapy. A Japanese study examining lymphatic flow before and after surgery found that compression garments can help reverse lymphoedema and restore lymphatic function for many patients, particularly if the lymphoedema is detected early (Akita, 2016).

Compression garments are typically used for long-term management once your lymphoedema swelling has stabilised. These garments are designed to apply graduated pressure to the arm, hand, breast or chest to help move fluid through your lymphatic vessels.

With guidance from a qualified lymphoedema therapist, you will be able to find a product that is suitable for you. It's important to choose the appropriate pressure level (or "class"), fabric and style, and to follow specific recommendations from your therapist, as well as the manufacturer's instructions, on when and how often to wear the garment. Let's explore these considerations in more detail on the following pages.

CLASS – PRESSURE LEVELS OF COMPRESSION GARMENTS

Compression garments are divided into classes based on how firm the fabric is on the skin. The amount of pressure is measured in millimetres of mercury (mmHg), similar to a blood pressure cuff. The higher the class, the more compression the garment can provide to treat your lymphoedema. Garments range from low pressure (class 1) to high pressure (class 4). The exact definition of each class varies by region, and sometimes within regions (see **Table 8.1**). The most commonly used definition is the German RAL standard.

For each class, the amount of pressure is given as a range (e.g. 23–32mmHg). The two levels in this range refer to the gradient of pressure applied along a limb. The lower level is the minimum force exerted at the widest part of the limb, such as around your shoulder or thigh, while the upper pressure is the maximum force applied at the narrowest part, like your wrist or ankle. This gradient moving from higher to lower pressure (e.g. wrist to shoulder, ankle to thigh) improves circulation by gently pushing blood and lymphatic fluid up the limb towards your heart, preventing fluid build-up and effectively reducing swelling.

ATTRIBUTE	Class 1	Class 2	Class 3	Class 4
Compression intensity	Low	Medium	High	Very High
Available ready-to-wear	Yes	Yes	Yes	No
Available custom-made	Yes	Yes	Yes	Yes
COMPRESSION PRESSURE STANDARD BY REGION* (mmHg)				
RAL	18–21	23–32	34–46	>49
French	10–15	15–20	20–36	>36
US	15–21	23–32	34–46	≥49
British	14–17	18–24	25–35	Not reported

*The RAL Quality Mark for Medical Compression Stockings (RAL-GZ-387/2) is the standard set by the German Institute for Quality Assurance and Certification. For the US standard, see reference USMCA (2018). There is no specific Australian standard.

Table 8.1
Comparison of compression classes and standards.

Compression pressure standards vary internationally and also depend on whether the garment is for an arm or leg. Take care when ordering garments without professional help (Todd, 2015; Scheer, 2017). This is something best done following a clinical assessment by a qualified therapist.

This assessment determines the level of compression that's best for you based on the specifics of your condition, such as the extent, stage and location of the swelling. Generally, a higher pressure level is recommended for managing more significant swelling, particularly in the legs. Legs typically require stronger compression than arms due to their larger volume and the added challenge of gravity, which causes fluid to pool and worsen swelling. Once the therapist has a clear understanding of your swelling – whether it is early or advanced, the areas it affects, and if there's any hand involvement – they will work with you to choose the most suitable class, fabric and style for your garment.

FABRIC – CIRCULAR-KNIT VERSUS FLAT-KNIT

Compression garments can be classified as circular-knit or flat-knit. The difference between the two types of garments is shown in **Table 8.2**. Circular-knit garments are mass-produced to fit standard sizes and are less expensive than custom-made, flat-knit garments. They are quicker to obtain and are designed to fit the regular anatomy of an arm or leg, but they may not fit you perfectly and can roll down at the top. Circular-knit garments are better for stage 0 (subclinical lymphoedema) or stage 1 (early lymphoedema), provided that you fit into the manufacturers' predefined size ranges.

A flat-knit garment is shaped to follow the contours of your body, creating a custom fit; the sides are joined together by a flat elastic seam. The main difference between flat-knit and circular-knit garments is the level of stiffness and compression they provide. Flat-knit garments offer more stiffness and a stronger outer structure, meaning they won't cut into soft tissues and can bridge over skin folds, which is particularly helpful for more severe lymphoedema. Circular-knit garments are made from thinner, more flexible material, so they tend to crease and press into skin folds. They don't provide the same firm outer structure as flat-knit garments, making them less effective for managing severe swelling.

FEATURE	CIRCULAR-KNIT GARMENT	FLAT-KNIT GARMENT
Product type	Ready-to-wear	Custom-made
Construction	Knitted on a circular machine, shaped by varying yarn tension and stitch height	Knitted on a flatbed machine, shaped by adjusting the number of stitches
Seam	Seamless, as it is knitted in a continuous circular process	Has a seam, as it is sewn together after knitting
Thickness	Generally thinner and lighter	Typically thicker, due to larger gauge needles
Stiffness	Lower stiffness, less containment	Higher stiffness, offering more containment
Customisation	Usually pre-made in standard sizes, some custom options available	Easily customisable to any shape
Application	Best for limbs with regular shapes, cosmetically more appealing	Better for limbs with irregular shapes, can bridge skin folds
Comfort	Usually more comfortable, due to lower stiffness and thinner fabric	Although higher stiffness might cause some pressure, a custom-made design generally ensures a better overall fit and comfort
Durability	May experience more wear and tear due to thinner fabric	More durable due to thicker fabric
Uses	Suitable for milder cases of lymphoedema requiring less compression and structural support	Recommended for more advanced cases of lymphoedema that need greater compression and support
Cost	Less expensive, especially in ready-to-wear options	Usually more expensive due to custom fitting and thicker materials
Pressure	Available in a wide range of pressure classes, though often used in lower to moderate ranges	Available in a wide range of pressure classes, from low to high
Colour	More colour options, including fashion styles	Limited colour options, usually neutral (beige, black, white, navy, red)

Table 8.2

Comparison of circular-knit and flat-knit compression garments.

STYLE – TYPES OF COMPRESSION GARMENTS

Lymphoedema varies from person to person, and there are several types of garments available to suit various patient needs. When we think about style, this includes the function of the garment, options for accessibility and, of course, the appearance.

Garment selection

When choosing the appropriate compression garment, your therapist will consider the location and stage of your lymphoedema. They will aim to find a style that extends beyond the swollen area to ensure optimal support, prevent fluid accumulation at the edges, and provide a comfortable fit. Examples of compression garments for upper limb lymphoedema include:

- Full-length sleeves combined with a gauntlet or glove, either separate (**Figure 8.1A**) or combined (**Figure 8.1B**)
- Shorter sleeves from wrist to axilla (**Figure 8.1C**)
- Fingerless gauntlets (**Figure 8.2A**)
- Gloves (extending to the fingers but not covering the fingertips) (**Figure 8.2B**).

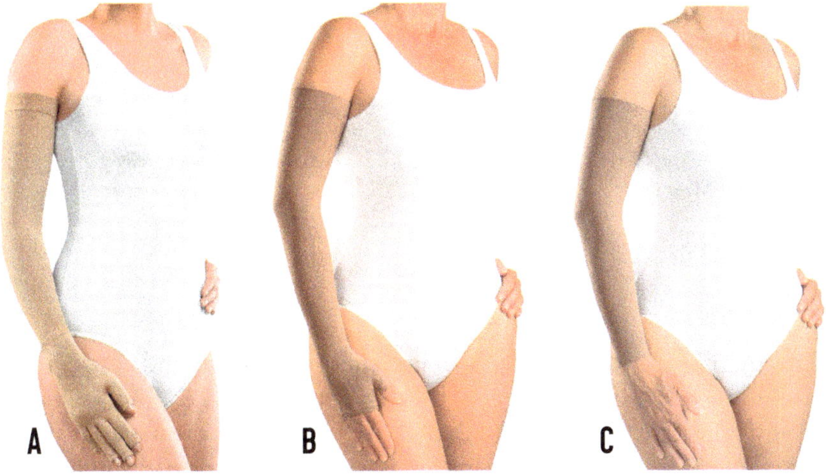

Figure 8.1

Compression garment types – A: sleeve (wrist to axilla) with separate glove, B: combined sleeve and glove, C: sleeve (wrist to axilla). Copyright Medi Australia, with permission.

Popular brands of compression garments include, in alphabetical order, Haddenham, Jobst, Juzo, LympheDIVAs, Medi and Solaris. The Australasian Lymphology Association provides a list of Australian suppliers on their website: visit https://www.lymphoedema.org.au/education-&-resources/lymphoedema-supplier-list/ (or see **Useful websites**, page 174).

Compression garments can be very expensive, but some governments offer compression garment schemes and subsidies. Some health insurance companies also cover part of the cost. Your lymphoedema therapist will be able to advise you about this.

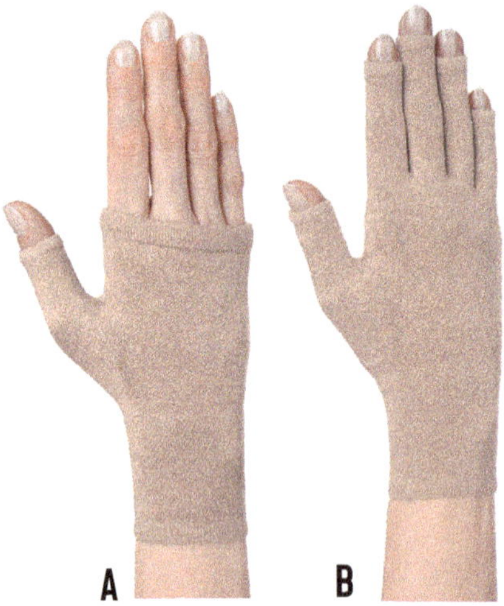

Figure 8.2

Compression garment types –
A: gauntlet, B: glove.
Copyright Medi Australia, with permission.

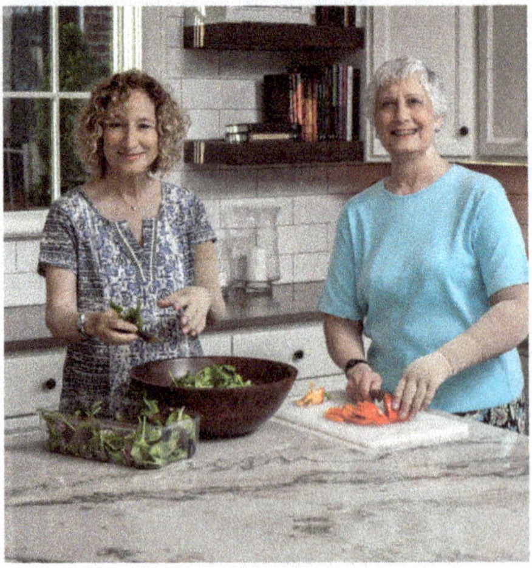

Figure 8.3

Example of a ready-to-wear compression garment. Copyright Essity, with permission.

Garment fit

Ready-to-wear

Ready-to-wear compression garments are an accessible and convenient solution when dealing with subclinical or early-stage lymphoedema causing minimal or mild swelling. These garments come in various pre-established sizes and compression levels, which makes them an immediate and straightforward option. They are also called off-the-shelf, ready-made or over-the-counter garments (**Figure 8.3**). Ready-to-wear garments still need to be prescribed by an accredited lymphoedema therapist.

Custom-made

Custom-made garments are particularly important when there is distortion of the limb shape; sometimes as a result of uneven swelling, the limb no longer follows its normal shape. In this case, you need a custom-made garment to be able to provide graduated compression to the limb. These made-to-measure garments are flat-knit and crafted to your individual requirements. If you have a larger, softer limb, a custom-made garment is generally recommended to ensure an optimal fit.

Adjustable compression wraps

Adjustable Velcro-type garments (see **Figure 6.5**) have gained prominence as a user-friendly option. Brands like Haddenham, Jobst, Juzo, Medi and Solaris offer leg and arm wraps with Velcro closures, allowing you to easily customise the level of compression. This adaptability allows for comfort, and these wraps are also practical as they generally need less assistance than conventional garments. (It's still best to have help to put these on, particularly for arm swelling.) These products are used more often for legs than arms, but are another option to consider in your lymphoedema therapist's toolkit.

Keep in mind that these wraps are bulkier than standard compression garments and require some skill to apply the correct level of compression. You might also consider adding zips to custom-made compression garments. Zips can make it easier to take the garments off, but you'll need good hand dexterity to put them on, and having someone to help you is advised.

Garment appearance

Depending on the manufacturer, compression garments come in flesh-tone colours such as beige, ivory, tan or brown; neutral colours such as white or black; bold colours such as pink, purple or red; or more colourful styles and fashion prints (**Figures 8.4–8.5**). Skin tones are the most common type selected by most patients, as they can make the garment feel more subtle.

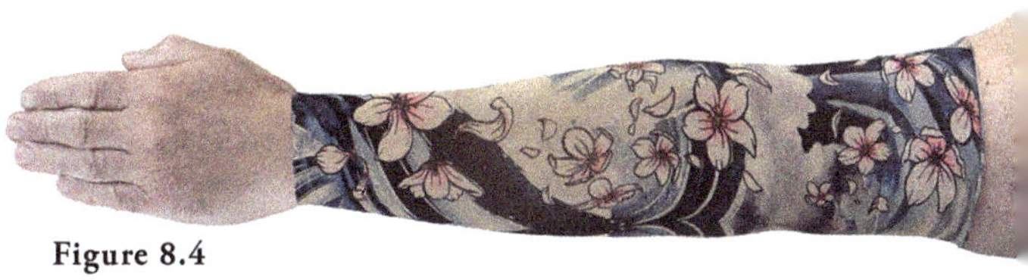

Figure 8.4

A creative compression garment from LympheDIVAs. Copyright LympheDIVAs LLC, with permission.

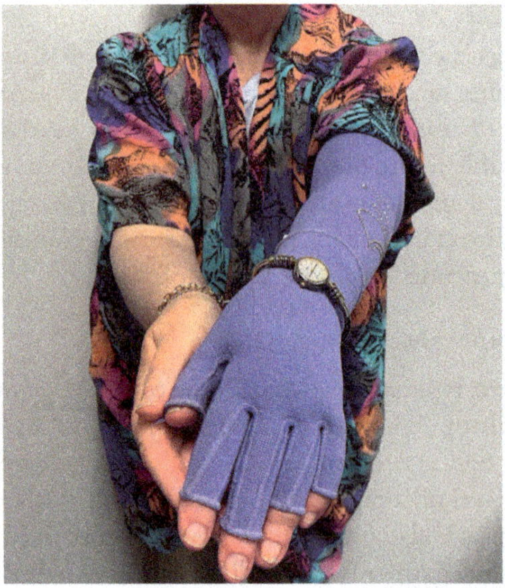

Figure 8.5

A flat-knit, custom-made compression sleeve (wrist to axilla) with separate glove made by Medi. The garment has a functional elbow zone and silicone top band.

WHAT DO I NEED TO LOOK FOR IN A COMPRESSION GARMENT?

When you are choosing a compression garment, there are some important points to keep in mind:

- Your garment should be comfortable, so see a lymphoedema therapist to have your sleeve properly measured and fitted. If you are buying a ready-to-wear garment, make sure you have it fitted by someone with experience.
- Your garment should have the right amount of pressure, depending on whether your lymphoedema is mild or more severe (see **Table 8.1**). It's like being prescribed a specific compression dose by your therapist. Check with your therapist class of garment they recommend; for arms, we generally don't use garments above class 2.
- Check with your therapist about whether you should wear a handpiece – a gauntlet **(Figure 8.2A)** or glove **(Figure 8.2B)** on your hand.

- You will need to replace your garment every six to nine months, as they stretch over time and lose compression. It's a good idea to set a reminder every six months to be refitted for a new garment.

Day and night garments

There are different types of garments for wearing during the day and at night. It is not usually recommended to wear daytime garments to bed, as they may be uncomfortable and cut into your skin. There are specific night-time garments available that are softer and have less compression. However, this is an extra expense that you may prefer to avoid. As a rule, if your swelling worsens overnight then you need to wear compression overnight. How you do this is an individual choice based on your clinical needs and personal preference. Work with your therapist to decide whether to wear your daytime garment to bed or try a lower-class night-time compression garment (see **Figures 6.6** and **10.3**).

OTHER TIPS FOR USING A COMPRESSION GARMENT

- Avoid applying moisturiser immediately before putting on your garment, as the chemicals may affect its durability. Use moisturiser when you take the garment off at night. Some compression companies may have special types of moisturisers that are less damaging to the garment material; check with your lymphoedema therapist.
- Putting on and taking off compression garments can be challenging. There are various devices available from medical supply companies to make this easier; ask your therapist for more information.
- You may like to wear a pair of household rubber gloves to help you put on your garment more easily.
- If you have an infection, such as cellulitis, you can wear your garment when it is comfortable to do so. Compression has, in fact, been shown to help reduce the incidence of cellulitis (Webb, 2020).
- If your garment cuts into your skin at various points, your therapist may add extra padding material to redistribute the pressure, or prescribe a garment of stiffer material.

- If you find you are gaining weight, or that your lymphoedema is getting worse, make an appointment with your therapist to recheck the fit of your garment.

The most important thing is to wear your garment consistently. No matter how perfectly it fits or how well made it is, if you don't actually wear your garment then it can't help you. If your garment is uncomfortable or causing a negative reaction, you're less likely to wear it, which means it won't be able to provide the positive compression benefits you need.

HOW LONG SHOULD I WEAR MY COMPRESSION GARMENT EACH DAY?

There is limited research on the most effective garment-wearing regimen. However, for most patients, the usual practice is to take the compression garment off at night. A simple approach is to put your garment on when you get dressed and take it off before or after dinner. You may end up wearing it for 10 to 12 hours a day or more, depending on the severity of your lymphoedema. Work with your therapist who will align your individual goals with the class, fabric and style of the compression garment. The approach should be tailored to you and how your lymphoedema responds to compression.

For patients with advanced lymphoedema (stage 2 or 3), it is a good idea to wear your compression garment 24 hours a day. Constant (24/7) compression is also advised for patients who have undergone liposuction (see **Chapter 10**, Liposuction for Lymphoedema). Once you are well and truly into the maintenance phase of your lymphoedema care, you can work with your therapist to determine a personalised compression plan that works for you. This will be a balance between your clinical needs, treatment goals and response to compression.

You may want to give night-time compression a try, in consultation with your therapist. One randomised controlled trial divided 120 patients with mild or moderate arm lymphoedema (from previous breast cancer) into three groups: the first group used daytime compression only, the second added night-time bandaging, and the third used a night-time compression support garment, or NCSG (McNeely, 2022). The researchers measured arm swelling over 12 weeks and found that adding compression at night, whether with bandaging or a garment, significantly reduced arm swelling compared to daytime-only compression. The groups using night-time compression showed a 12% decrease in arm swelling with bandaging and a 16% decrease with an NCSG, compared to a 1.5% reduction of swelling in the standard care group.

Interestingly, the benefit was more pronounced in participants with mild lymphoedema, who responded better to night-time compression than those with moderate lymphoedema. This may be because moderate to severe cases involve more fatty tissue and fibrosis, which reduces the effectiveness of compression. All participants reported improved quality of life, irrespective of their group allocation.

The study concluded that adding night-time compression is a valuable strategy for managing lymphoedema. An accompanying editorial by Cheryl Brunelle and Alphonse Taghian provides a great overview of the subject (Brunelle, 2022); however, you should still talk to your lymphoedema therapist before starting night-time compression.

HOW DO I PUT ON AND TAKE OFF MY GARMENT?

It is vital that you can easily don and doff your compression garment to use it safely. Improper garment handling can damage both the garment and your skin, and it can impair your circulation. Ask your lymphoedema therapist to help you put on and take off your garment to check and advise on your technique.

Some devices are available at extra cost to help with donning and doffing. As mentioned earlier, rubber gloves may be enough to provide the extra friction you need to handle your garment. Do not fold over the top or bottom of your garment to fit; instead, smooth the garment out to remove any wrinkles and redistribute the material across your arm or leg. If you are not confident with this process, see your therapist for more guidance.

HOW DO I LOOK AFTER MY GARMENT?

Compression garments are expensive, so looking after them will save you time and money in the long run. Most therapists advise that you have at least two garments – one to wear and one in the wash. Make sure you follow the manufacturer's instructions for washing the garment. Washing it in a delicates bag or pillowcase can also help protect it in the washing machine. Daily washing will remove any sweat, germs and dry skin, and help the garment to retain its compression which makes it last longer.

To dry your garment, lay it flat on a towel or between two towels, away from sunlight or direct heat. Most manufacturers advise against using the spin cycle on your washing machine or using a tumble dryer; be sure to check the instructions for your particular garment. Do not iron your garment.

HOW OFTEN SHOULD I BUY A NEW GARMENT?

When you first start wearing a garment, your lymphoedema therapist will measure you every few months to ensure the fit is correct. You will need to keep replacing the garments regularly over time – I usually recommend getting a new garment every six months, but this frequency may increase if your condition changes or your garment is losing its stretch.

Replacing compression garments can be very expensive, but it's an important part of treatment, as a poorly fitted or worn out garment won't help your lymphoedema.

Professor Håkan Brorson explains: "Managing lymphoedema is comparable to managing diabetes. Just as insulin is essential for keeping blood sugar levels within a normal range, compression garments are necessary to prevent the accumulation of oedema. Prescribing only one vial of insulin per year when a patient requires 12 would be unthinkable, and the same principle applies to compression garments. One garment per year is not sufficient if eight are needed. In many countries, patients face limits of one or two garments per year, forcing them to pay out-of-pocket for additional ones, which jeopardises treatment success. In contrast, Nordic countries have no restrictions on the number of garments prescribed, leading to better treatment outcomes."

COMPRESSION GARMENTS AND INTIMACY

It's normal for compression garments to affect your body image – a lot of patients say that wearing a garment makes them feel "less sexy". No doubt, having a supportive partner will reduce your anxiety about your lymphoedema. Don't hesitate to remove your garment for intimacy if that is your preferred approach. Although consistent compression is essential, spending some time without your garment is also OK.

Some of my patients take their garment off if they are going out for a special occasion. Be flexible as you get to know your new body – your garment should fit in with your lifestyle, not the other way around. However, this may not always be possible. It's important to listen to your body and pay attention to your lymphoedema. If you find that removing your garment causes the swelling to reaccumulate rapidly, then it's best to keep the breaks to a minimum.

WHAT DO I DO IF COMPRESSION IS NOT WORKING?

Compression garments need updating and adjusting from time to time. Your therapist may need to change the garment measurements or add extra padding over pressure areas. Sometimes they may need to start the measurement and fitting process again. If compression is not working for you, I would recommend an assessment by a multidisciplinary lymphoedema team, which includes lymphoedema therapists, doctors and possibly surgeons. You may need some imaging to look beneath the skin. It is possible that your lymphoedema has progressed to become more fatty, as discussed in **Chapter 2**, What Is Lymphoedema?

If your arm hurts or is numb, or you have new pins and needles, see your therapist urgently for another assessment, as your garment is likely not a good fit. If the pain continues or if you notice sudden swelling in a limb, it's important to see your family doctor, surgeon or oncologist for reassessment. This may include getting imaging such as an MRI, CT or **PET-CT scan**. If there's a chance that you have deep vein thrombosis, an urgent venous Doppler test is needed.

9

OTHER LYMPHOEDEMA THERAPIES

LASER THERAPY

Laser therapy has been used to treat lymphoedema for many years. Lymphoedema is one of several conditions that respond to this therapy, including arthritis, inflammation of the tendons and carpal tunnel syndrome (which can occur after hormonal treatments for breast cancer).

There are other terms for this approach, including photobiomodulation therapy (PBMT), low-power laser, and **low-level laser therapy** (LLLT). I usually refer to it as "laser therapy" for simplicity. Laser therapy is a non-invasive treatment that uses low-level lasers or light-emitting diodes (LEDs) to stimulate healing and reduce inflammation. It is different from the high-level lasers used to cut or destroy tissue during surgery.

In 1967, Professor Endre Mester at Semmelweis University in Hungary applied what he thought was high-powered laser energy to implanted tumours on the backs of mice, and found that it stimulated hair growth but left the tumours unchanged. Initially baffled, he discovered that his laser device was wrongly emitting a low rather than high level of power. His later experiments found that this low-power laser therapy stimulated wound healing (Gáspár, 2009).

The mechanism by which laser therapy works is not fully understood. It is thought to increase energy production by the **mitochondria** in the cells of the body. This increase in energy can help to stimulate healing and reduce inflammation, which may improve lymphoedema symptoms. There is also research to suggest that laser therapy encourages the production of new lymphatic vessels and improves lymphatic circulation (Karu, 2007).

Laser therapy for lymphoedema typically involves placing a handheld device over the affected area for 20 to 30 minutes. It does not cause the tissue to heat up, and most patients don't feel anything when the treatment is given. There is mixed evidence to support laser therapy as an effective treatment for lymphoedema. A meta-analysis conducted by Mahmood (2022) looked at how laser therapy could help with breast cancer-related swelling after surgery, reviewing a selection of studies published since 2010. The researchers found that laser therapy reduced the swelling, but did not significantly improve shoulder movement or pain compared to **placebo** treatments with no laser.

Nevertheless, there have been marked improvements in laser technology since these earlier studies were done. Baxter (2017) documented the evolution

of the various laser therapies used for lymphoedema. The original hand-held lasers were called category 1, or class 1. They have longer treatment times and do not penetrate deeply into the tissues. There are now several laser devices available, ranging from the original class 1 (5W) devices to the latest hands-free class 4 (75W) devices with robotised scanning.
Several differences exist between class 1 and class 4 lasers, including treatment time. Class 4 lasers are five times faster, taking 18 seconds to treat a small trigger point compared with 100 seconds to deliver the same dose using a class 1 laser. While there hasn't been research to officially compare class 4 lasers against the earlier models, I've heard very positive feedback from lymphoedema therapists and patients vouching for their effectiveness.

One class 4 laser, known as the MLS (multiwave locked system) laser, emits light in red and infrared wavelengths and can penetrate up to 5cm beneath the skin (**Figure 9.1**). Unlike surgical lasers, which typically penetrate only a few millimetres to ensure precise cutting of tissue, the MLS laser uses a combination of continuous and pulsed light for non-invasive deep tissue therapy.

Therapists can utilise a hands-free component, the "Charlie head", with three laser diodes for treating larger areas, or add a hand-held device for simultaneous treatment of two regions. For example, the Charlie head can target breast oedema while the hand-held component works on lymphoedema in the arm.

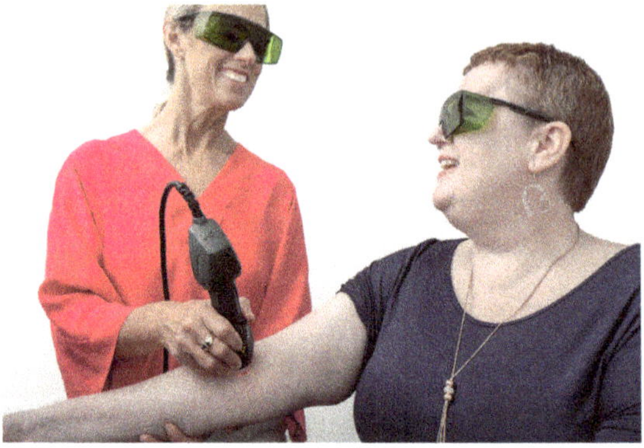

Figure 9.1

A Multiwave Locked System (MLS) laser therapy device.
Both the operator and the patient wear protective glasses during the treatment (https://lymphaticsolutions.com.au/services/mls-laser-therapy).

KINESIOLOGY TAPING

Kinesiology taping (KT) has been used in sports medicine for many years. It involves placing a one-way stretch tape along swollen parts of the body. For arm lymphoedema, therapists often use it to support lymphatic flow between weekly manual lymphatic drainage treatments. The tape works by lifting the skin and providing more space for the accumulated lymphatic fluid to move towards the axilla (see **Figure 9.2**).

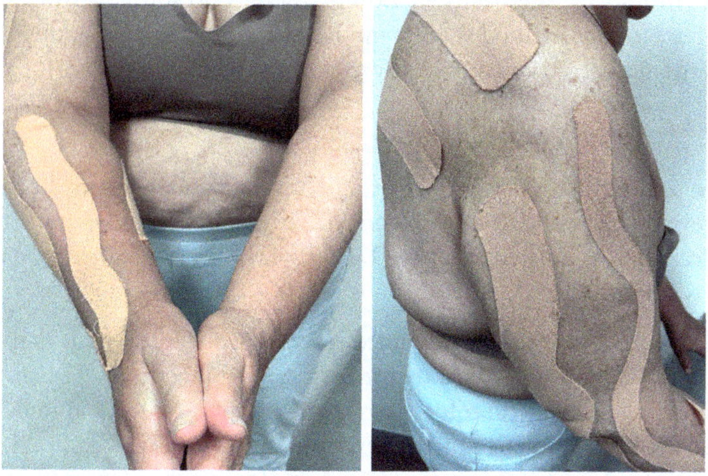

Figure 9.2

Kinesiology taping (KT) for arm and hand lymphoedema.

There has been some research done on the efficacy of kinesiology tape. In one study from Spain, 30 patients with chronic breast cancer-related lymphoedema were given four weeks of compression therapy and four weeks of KT, with a four-week gap before each intervention as a washout period (Otero, 2019). The study found that four weeks of KT was more effective than four weeks of wearing a compression garment.

During KT therapy, the participants had a significant reduction in arm volume and a better quality of life; their symptoms of pain, tightness, heaviness and hardness all improved, they had better mobility in the affected limb, and they found the taping to be more comfortable. The authors noted that extreme caution is required when removing the tape to avoid skin tears, and that the total duration of treatment should be limited to a maximum of four weeks. Skin allergy to the tape is also a rare complication (Otero, 2019).

In a recent meta-analysis of 14 randomised controlled trials of KT for over 500 patients, the authors found that although taping did not reduce the severity of lymphoedema, it did significantly improve upper limb function, quality of life, and perceived comfort (Yang, 2024). I've had many patients who have benefitted from KT – it's particularly helpful in areas that are hard to compress, like the hand, or the shoulder underneath wrapping. There is no simple answer as to which treatment method is best, and it's often a matter of working with your therapist to try various options and see what works best for you.

MEDICAL TREATMENTS FOR LYMPHOEDEMA

There has been research into treating lymphoedema with medication. However, while some treatments can relieve lymphoedema symptoms, no medical interventions have emerged as a magic bullet to effectively manage or cure the condition.

A recent systematic review examined several small clinical trials that had investigated various medical treatments for lymphoedema. The studies explored selenium, ketoprofen, benzopyrones, doxycycline and stem-cell therapies, but no standout treatment was identified (Walker, 2022). In general, you should avoid medical treatments for lymphoedema unless you are part of a clinical trial.

Diuretics

The basic mechanism of **diuretics** is to stimulate your kidneys to produce more urine, removing excess fluid from the body. However, diuretics primarily target fluid in the circulatory system (bloodstream) rather than the fluid in the interstitium (tissues). This includes lymph, which accumulates due to lymphatic dysfunction in lymphoedema. While diuretics may seem like a helpful way to reduce swelling, they are not effective at removing protein-rich lymphatic fluid from your tissues and may inadvertently worsen lymphoedema. Additionally, diuretics can disturb the body's electrolyte balance, causing issues like low potassium. Although diuretics are used to treat fluid retention caused by heart failure, patients with lymphoedema should avoid them. An exception might be if your doctor prescribes you a temporary course of diuretics for another medical condition.

Nonsteroidal anti-inflammatory drugs

Nonsteroidal anti-inflammatory drugs (NSAIDs) can help to reduce inflammation and improve lymphatic function. However, most studies involving NSAIDs are small, and they have not been found to effectively treat lymphoedema. NSAIDs work by inhibiting the production of prostaglandins, which are molecules that play a role in inflammation and pain.

Professor Stanley Rockson is a pre-eminent leader in lymphoedema treatment and a dedicated clinician. He has spent a good part of his career studying various drug treatments for lymphoedema; in one of his early trials, he found that an NSAID called ketoprofen reduced skin thickening associated with lymphoedema. While favourable responses to ketoprofen are encouraging, the widespread, chronic use of ketoprofen is limited, as with all NSAIDs, by a "black box warning" regarding cardiovascular toxicity (Rockson, 2018).

Corticosteroids

Corticosteroids are more potent anti-inflammatory drugs that work by suppressing the immune system. While these drugs can be effective at reducing swelling and inflammation, they also have unpleasant side effects such as weight gain, stomach ulcers, high blood pressure and increased risk of infection. They have not been very effective in treating lymphoedema.

Other medical treatments

Benzopyrones, derived from naturally occurring substances, are used to manage oedema that is high in protein by promoting the breakdown and removal of proteins in the lymphatic fluid. However, the clinical effectiveness of benzopyrones (including compounds like diosmin and hesperidin) remains uncertain, and they are not considered a primary treatment for lymphoedema.

Acupuncture

A systematic review by Chien (2019) evaluated the effect of acupuncture on breast cancer-related lymphoedema across six different trials involving 178 patients. This review aimed to determine the safety and effectiveness of acupuncture as a complementary therapy. While acupuncture was found to be safe, with none of the trials reporting any major complications, its impact on reducing arm circumference in patients did not reach statistical significance. However, some individual studies within the review indicated potential symptom improvement, such as reduced pain and better quality of life, suggesting that acupuncture may be beneficial for some patients. The authors concluded that more randomised controlled trials are needed, on a larger scale, to confirm these findings and better understand the benefits of acupuncture for breast cancer-related lymphoedema.

Brenda's Story

I had breast cancer that was treated in 2015 with a lumpectomy and radiation therapy. I was in hospital having investigations when my arm and hand became swollen, seven years after treatment.

I tried a full-length arm compression garment, which did not work, and then a glove and sleeve, which caused swelling in my wrist. We then tried using a garment for the arm alone, but that caused swelling in my hand.

My lymphoedema therapist decided to try some taping, and I couldn't believe that my hand had returned to normal overnight. I have now been having taping for two weeks without a sleeve, taping my whole arm and around to my back. Taping certainly has worked for me.

John's Story

I worked for over 15 years with a wonderful lymphoedema therapist, Louise Koelmeyer, an international leader in this field. We started together at the Westmead Breast Cancer Institute, where I began funding her early detection program for lymphoedema using bioimpedance spectroscopy (BIS).

Initially, I was a bit sceptical about the BIS early detection program, but soon realised that our patients loved it. They liked the reassurance of a normal test or the feedback they received if their fluid levels begin to rise.

In the early years, Louise often teased me for calling it by the wrong name. "John, it's not M-Dex! Think of lymphoedema, or Louise!" she would say with despair as she drummed "L-Dex" into me.

These days, I am convinced that BIS will be used even more over time, to measure not just lymphoedema but our bones, heart function, and fat and muscle composition, helping many patients with cancer and other chronic diseases on their way to recovery.

When I moved to Macquarie University in 2011, I convinced Louise to join me, and together we established the Australian Lymphoedema Education, Research and Treatment (ALERT) Centre. In 2020, ALERT was awarded a prestigious "Center of Excellence" designation by the US-based Lymphatic Education and Research Network (see **Useful websites**, page 174).

10

LIPOSUCTION FOR LYMPHOEDEMA

When I first started the ALERT Centre in 2012, Dr Helen Mackie approached me looking for a plastic surgeon to perform liposuction on one of her patients.

Dr Mackie has dedicated her career to helping patients with lymphoedema. Lymphoedema is a specialty developed through clinical experience, and lymphoedema specialists come from a variety of backgrounds; Dr Mackie is a rehabilitation specialist, and others are cardiologists, dermatologists, plastic surgeons or radiation oncologists like me. These exceptional individuals make it their mission to treat patients with this challenging condition, and they have my full respect.

Until I worked with Dr Mackie, I had never heard of liposuction for lymphoedema. As an oncologist, I was trained to be cautious with needles when taking blood, let alone inserting even bigger needles into the arm! I also had no idea that lymphoedema stimulated fat production.

Before long, Dr Mackie and my deputy, A/Prof Louise Koelmeyer, had shown me the evidence on liposuction and found an international expert, Dr Alex Munnoch, who could train one of our surgical colleagues to perform the procedure. Dr Munnoch had been trained by Professor Brorson in 2004 and implemented the technique in Scotland. He trained Dr Thomas Lam, a plastic surgeon who worked with me in our breast cancer program. Dr Lam was a willing student and successfully performed liposuction on Dr Mackie's lymphoedema patient.

After the procedure, it was reported on the Channel 10 news in Sydney, and I remember the patient saying how pleased she was that she could put a coat on for the first time in many years. It's these little things that we take for granted that make life very difficult for patients with lymphoedema. Some of my patients have travelled overseas, at great expense, to have their clothes specially tailored for their asymmetrical limbs. Further, the impact of a swollen limb on causing recurrent infections (cellulitis), often requiring time in hospital, is a nightmare. Liposuction has been found to reduce pain, reduce the incidence of cellulitis, and improve quality of life for patients with lymphoedema.

At the ALERT Centre, our team are extremely grateful to have learned from Professor Håkan Brorson, the "father of lymphoedema liposuction", from Skåne University Hospital in Malmö, Sweden. He took us under his wing, guided us through many complex cases, and welcomed our team to Sweden in 2013 where he gave them specialised training. One of the great honours of my career has been working with Professor Brorson and conducting lymphoedema research together.

Brorson's passion and leadership in this area has helped thousands of patients, despite the fact that his technique isn't technically a cure as it does not allow patients to stop wearing their compression garment. Yes, patients still have to wear a compression garment after liposuction, but they can also wear regular clothes, improve their fitness and spend less time in hospital with cellulitis (Brorson, 2012). Liposuction can be used for both arm and leg lymphoedema (see Jayne's story, page 106 and Sharne's story, page 107).

HOW DO I KNOW IF I'M ELIGIBLE FOR LIPOSUCTION?

Liposuction is suitable for more advanced lymphoedema (stage 2B or 3), where the lymphatic fluid in your affected limb has become replaced with fatty tissue. To be considered for liposuction, you must have tried complex lymphoedema therapy (CLT), including manual lymphatic drainage and compression therapy performed by a skilled lymphoedema therapist. CLT is performed until pitting has disappeared or there is minimal pitting (no more than 3–4mm). As discussed in **Chapter 2**, What Is Lymphoedema?, the pitting test involves pressing firmly into the swelling for at least 60 seconds to see if the pressure causes indentation (see **Figure 2.3**). If you still have swelling after conservative treatment with CLT, and there is minimal or no pitting, liposuction can be performed to remove the excess fat. An MRI scan is often done to confirm the amount of fat versus fluid in your swollen arm or leg (see **Figures 2.2** and **4.9**).

It is important to emphasise that liposuction will not "cure" your lymphoedema, but will treat the secondary effect of fat accumulation. Removing the fat will help your limb return to its usual size and improve its mobility and function.

Below are the ALERT Centre's selection criteria for liposuction, which we developed in conjunction with Professor Håkan Brorson.

You are eligible for liposuction if you have:

- Late-stage lymphoedema with fatty changes and minimal fluid in the limb
- A percentage limb volume difference between the affected and unaffected side of 20% or more. (This difference may be as low as 10% in some patients.) At ALERT, the average limb volume difference was 42%, falling to a 2% difference five years after liposuction (Karlsson, 2024).

- Problems with function in the affected limb, such as impaired mobility, that require intervention
- No recent cellulitis (infection)
- No skin lesions or ulcers on the affected limb
- No evidence of active cancer
- No surgical or anaesthetic contraindications for liposuction.

You also need to:

- Have completed and complied with conservative treatment, including massage, bandaging and wearing of firm compression garments
- Be willing and committed to undergo regular follow-up, wear your compression garments day and night (except for shower ing), and replace the garments as needed.

HOW DOES LIPOSUCTION WORK?

Liposuction involves removing fat via 15–20 small incisions (5mm each) along the arm or leg. The treatment is effective because it removes the excess fatty tissue; it is nearly 100% successful in reducing the girth and weight of a patient's arm and reducing the incidence of severe infection (cellulitis). There is a complete reduction of swelling, which decreases symptoms of pain and heaviness and improves mobility. This volume reduction comes from both the surgery and the pre- and postoperative care from a lymphoedema therapist, with 24/7 use of a custom-made compression garment. The arm usually matches the unaffected side within six months, and the results continue long-term – in **Figure 10.1** below, the "after" picture was taken six years after liposuction.

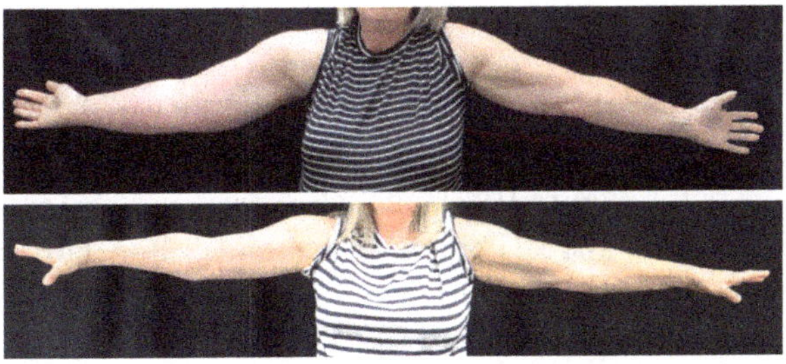

Figure 10.1

Before (top image) and after (bottom) liposuction for advanced lymphoedema of the right arm. Preoperative volume difference was 1,333ml, meaning the right arm was 1.33kg heavier than the left. Copyright ALERT, Macquarie University, with permission.
See Jayne's story, page 106.

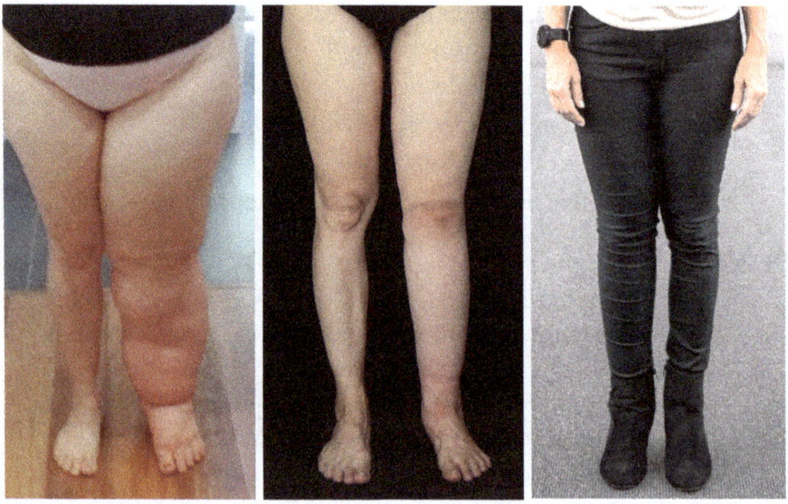

Figure 10.2

Severe left leg oedema following surgery to lymph nodes in the groin: before liposuction (left image), and 30 months later (middle and right) after treatment. See Sharne's story, page 107.

WILL LIPOSUCTION CURE MY LYMPHOEDEMA?

Unfortunately, liposuction surgery is not curative. Instead, it offers an opportunity to improve your limb function and overall quality of life while minimising the risk of lymphoedema progression.

In our cohort of lymphoedema patients from the ALERT Centre, we have seen very few complications from liposuction. Some patients have experienced skin damage from the postoperative garments, causing localised ulcers, but these tend to heal fairly quickly.

Our patients reported that pain, heaviness and swelling in the affected limb, as well as self-consciousness and anxiety, were all significantly improved after liposuction (see **Figure 10.2**). They also experienced fewer episodes of cellulitis (Schaverien, 2018). Long-term pre- and postoperative follow-up has shown that liposuction reduces the incidence of cellulitis by 87% for patients with arm lymphoedema (Lee, 2016) and by 65% for those with leg lymphoedema (Karlsson, 2022).

However, it is important to discuss liposuction with your specialist so that you fully understand the risks and benefits. There are potential complications of the procedure, including postoperative infection, bruising, skin necrosis, wound breakdown and blood clots. This is similar to any surgical procedure, but the risks are low. One common side effect of liposuction is numbness in the skin due to minor nerve damage; this usually goes away in a few weeks or months.

WHAT MANAGEMENT IS REQUIRED AFTER LIPOSUCTION?

Compression garments – postoperative care

Custom-made compression garments are created at least two weeks before your surgery, based on the dimensions of your limb on the unaffected side. One set of garments is applied after the procedure while you are still under anaesthetic. Two days after liposuction, these will be removed with the help of nursing staff so that you can shower; then the other garments are donned while the used set is washed and dried. This process is repeated every two days until you are discharged from hospital. You will be helped out of bed on the same day of your surgery to get you moving, with the help of some short-term pain relief.

Once you are home, you will alternate between two sets of compression garments (e.g. two sleeves and two gloves for arm lymphoedema), changing them every two days for the first week and then daily. Washing the garments daily helps to maintain the level of compression due to shrinkage in the wash (Brorson, 2012).

Compression garments – ongoing management

After liposuction, treatment continues with the use of constant compression. This is very important during the first three months after surgery, when the most notable changes in limb volume occur. New custom-made garments are required at the three-month follow-up visit after limb volume has decreased, and usually six and 12 months later.

Measuring garments after liposuction is a complex process that must be done by specially trained lymphoedema therapists. The sizing is calculated differently from that of a regular compression garment, requiring close collaboration between you and your therapist to achieve the best fit.

After complete limb volume reduction, you typically need to be checked every six months, when new garments are often prescribed. These garments will generally be the same size as your unaffected limb.

WHAT ARE THE SUCCESS RATES OF LIPOSUCTION?

As evidence of the long-term success of liposuction, Brorson (2015) published data from 146 breast cancer patients who underwent liposuction for arm lymphoedema and were followed up for 21 years. The results showed an average reduction in arm volume of 103% after three months, and more than 100% during the 21 years of follow-up. In other words, the treated arm was actually smaller than the healthy arm within three months of having liposuction, and this remained stable for over 20 years. Similar results were found for patients with leg lymphoedema (Brorson, 2022).

In our latest research from the ALERT Centre, we found that in patients with arm lymphoedema who underwent liposuction, the median preoperative volume difference between the affected and unaffected arm was 1061ml, which reduced to 79ml one year after surgery and 22ml five years after surgery (Karlsson, 2024). For patients with leg lymphoedema, the median volume difference was 3,447ml before liposuction; this reduced to 263ml one year after surgery, but went back up to 669ml at the five-year mark.

HOW DO I FIND THE RIGHT SURGICAL TEAM?

If you are considering surgical intervention such as liposuction, you will need the support of a comprehensive multidisciplinary team. The Lymphedema Education and Research Network (LE&RN) is an excellent place to start. On their website you can find a list of LE&RN "Centers of Excellence", which are institutions around the world considered expert in the multidisciplinary treatment and care of patients with lymphoedema and lymphatic diseases. (Visit https://lymphaticnetwork.org/centers-of-excellence or see **Useful websites**, page 174.)

It is important to approach all surgical treatments with caution. Don't rush into surgery; seek a second opinion if the results you are being quoted are too good to be true. Make sure you have taken an active part in a comprehensive program with a lymphoedema therapist prior to surgery, and that you are comfortable in your compression garments. In general, lymphoedema surgery is not advised in the first 6–12 months after cancer treatment.

MANAGING YOUR EXPECTATIONS

Choosing to have surgery for lymphoedema is a very difficult decision. It is important to think about your expectations and goals when considering all possible treatment options. Different surgical options or combinations of options exist, and have been reviewed elsewhere (Boyages, 2020; McGinity, 2024).

For some patients, their main priority is to reduce the time they spend wearing a compression garment; this cannot be achieved with liposuction. Some patients seek surgical intervention to minimise the possibility of future disease progression.

The lymphoedema staging classification may guide your choice of surgery. You also need the motivation to undergo a complicated procedure and maintain the necessary follow-up. Cost is a major consideration, as this type of surgery may not be covered by your health insurance or by Medicare.

Surgeons tend to be concerned about operating on patients who are obese or have significant medical illnesses, as this can increase the risk of postoperative surgical complications.

The main thing to remember when considering liposuction is that it won't cure your underlying lymphoedema, and you will need to continue with constant garment compression after the procedure. Many patients choose not to have liposuction for this reason alone. That doesn't mean you can't remove your garment for a special occasion, but leaving it off permanently will cause your lymphoedema to return.

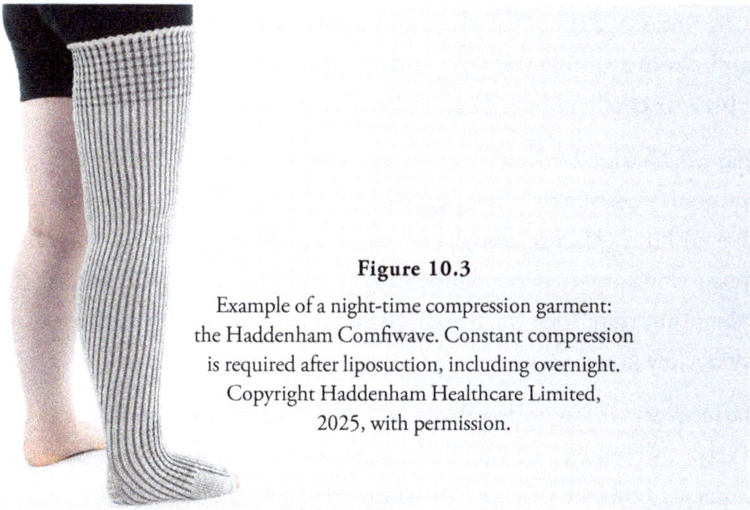

Figure 10.3

Example of a night-time compression garment: the Haddenham Comfiwave. Constant compression is required after liposuction, including overnight. Copyright Haddenham Healthcare Limited, 2025, with permission.

Jayne's Story

My story began in England, where I trained as a registered nurse before making a spontaneous decision to move to Australia in 1986. Life took a turn in 1991, when my husband and I moved to Singapore. Within weeks of arriving, I felt a lump in my breast. The diagnosis hit like a storm: breast cancer. I was shocked, but the care I received in Singapore was exceptional. I underwent a lumpectomy, axillary clearance, chemotherapy and radiotherapy. It was a surreal time; cancer was a taboo topic in Singapore, so I stood out in that regard, especially when I attended an awareness event with the prime minister.

After my treatment, I managed without lymphoedema for years, wearing only a light compression sleeve when needed. I raised two beautiful girls, breastfeeding them on one side, surprising even myself with how well we adapted.

It wasn't until 2016 that lymphoedema appeared. I was on holiday in England when my arm suddenly swelled up after a round of golf, and stayed swollen throughout the trip. Back in Australia, I sought help from a massage therapist, but nothing worked. My arm was heavy and cumbersome; simple tasks like turning over in bed or finding clothes that fit became challenging. My confidence crumbled.

That all changed when I was referred to the lymphoedema clinic at Macquarie University. The team were knowledgeable and supportive, and gave me hope. After thorough evaluations, including an MRI, I underwent liposuction surgery in September 2017. I was nervous but determined not to let it interfere with the rest of my life. I even timed my surgery around my hockey grand final!

The recovery was smoother than I expected. I stayed in hospital for a couple of days and wore my compression garments religiously. Five weeks post-surgery, I competed in the Australian Masters in Tasmania and won a

Jayne's Story cont'd

gold medal. My arm had slimmed down significantly, and my life was transformed. I no longer felt weighed down by my condition. I embraced tools like the ComfiSleeve and a lymphoedema pump, which I used every night, even while travelling.

The journey hasn't been without its challenges. I still experience occasional numbness and puffy shoulders, and I can't sleep comfortably on my right side. But the benefits far outweigh the inconveniences. I feel confident, capable and proud to compete in the sports I love – hockey, swimming and golf.

The team at the ALERT Centre gave me my life back, and I face every day with renewed hope and excitement for what's to come.

Sharne's Story

People would do double-takes when they saw me. It wasn't just a glance; it was the kind of look that made you want to shrink away and hide. That's why I started finding excuses to stay home, away from the stares and the questions.

It all started when I was diagnosed with cervical cancer. At the time, my youngest of six children was just two years old. I went through all the treatments – surgery, radiation, chemotherapy – determined to beat the disease. And I did. But what came afterwards was something I never expected. I developed secondary lymphoedema, and in many ways, it was worse than the cancer.

My left leg swelled up until it was 12.5kg heavier than my right. It was like carrying around a constant reminder of everything I'd been through, except this wasn't something I could conquer with a single treatment or

Sharne's Story cont'd

surgery. The swelling made it impossible to work full-time, move easily, or even wear normal shoes. I couldn't climb stairs, dress normally, or feel comfortable in my own skin. Sometimes, I wondered if I'd be better off without the leg altogether. I couldn't sit on the floor to be with the primary school students I was teaching.

Lymphoedema was more than just a physical burden; it was emotionally crippling. I felt isolated because no one really understood what I was going through. There was plenty of support during my cancer treatment, but lymphoedema? Hardly anyone talked about it. Even doctors didn't seem to know much about it, and I often felt dismissed or overlooked. My weight climbed to 115kg.

Then, I heard about liposuction surgery for lymphoedema at the ALERT Centre at Macquarie University. I was desperate for something to change, so I went for it.

I travelled from Yeppoon in Queensland – an eight-hour drive to Brisbane and then an hour's flight to Sydney. When I first walked into the ALERT clinic, I couldn't even climb the eight steps to the clinic door. But three months after the liposuction, I climbed the Sydney Harbour Bridge: 1,390 steps. I answered "no" to all the consent form questions; that's how much of a difference it made. I started working full-time again, travelling, and living the life I'd almost given up on.

Since my surgery, I have completed a single full marathon and run about 40 half-marathons, with training runs being around 30–50km per week, depending upon my training goal. I got my weight down to 64kg at the time of the marathon but now sit around 68kg. I enjoy family time with my six children and plenty of active time with my seven grandchildren.

I enjoy life without restriction, buying off-the-rack clothes and shoes,

Sharne's Story cont'd

travelling extensively and wearing my compression garment without any thought to what it stops me from doing. In fact, it feels strange without it!

It was an honour to have "the father of liposuction for lymphoedema", Håkan Brorson, together with the ALERT team, help me change my life.

Lymphoedema is still a part of my life, and I have to manage it, but now it doesn't define me. I feel like I've gotten my life back, and I am incredibly grateful for that.

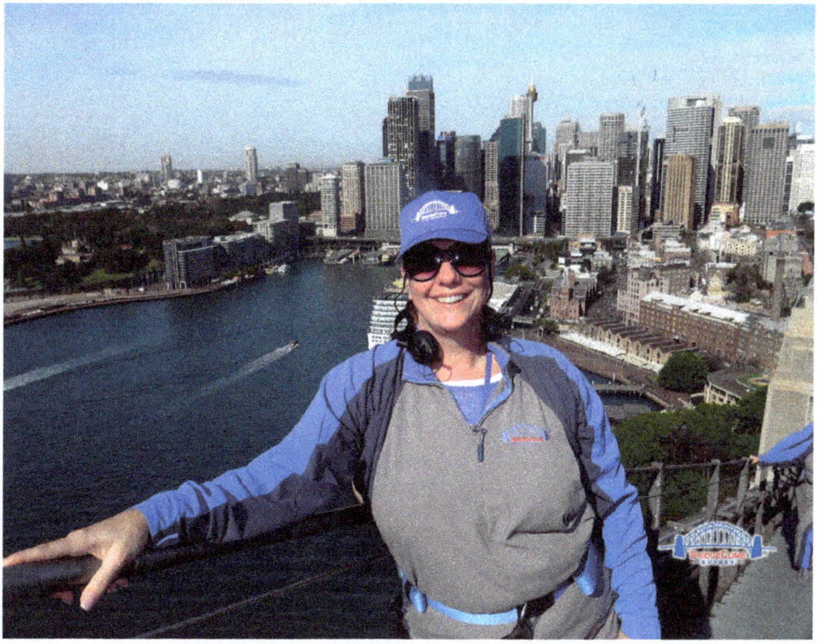

Figure 10.4

Sharne at the top of Sydney Harbour Bridge after climbing 1,390 steps!
Image supplied, with permission.

11

LYMPHATIC MICROSURGERY

LYMPHOVENOUS ANASTOMOSIS

You may recall from **Chapter 1**, Understanding the Lymphatic System, that the lymphatic system works closely with the cardiovascular system as they circulate blood and lymph around the body. Lymph is absorbed from body tissues, flows through a series of lymphatic vessels, and eventually empties into a large vein in the lower neck.

Some pioneering work in **lymphovenous anastomosis (LVA)** surgery was done at St Vincent's Hospital Melbourne in the 1970s (O'Brien, 1977). In the last 15 years we have seen more research in this area, due to advancements in imaging and surgical techniques, and more powerful microscopes. In 1997, a plastic surgeon in Japan reported performing "supermicrosurgery", connecting vessels of just 0.8mm diameter to tiny venules under the skin that were as small as 0.3mm (Koshima, 1998). This technique was later applied to patients with lymphoedema.

How does LVA work?

In LVA surgery, the surgeon connects a lymphatic vessel in the affected limb to a nearby tiny vein (called a **venule**) to bypass the damaged area and restore lymphatic circulation, so lymph can flow back into the bloodstream. The connection is called an **anastomosis**. LVA is also known as lymphovenous bypass (LVB). The procedure can be delayed (the most common approach) or immediate, where a bypass is done during axillary lymph node dissection.

A special vein-viewer is used to help locate the smaller venules. Indocyanine green (ICG) is injected before surgery to identify the damaged area and help the surgeon determine where the connections (anastomoses) will be made. It is also used during surgery to check whether the new links between the vessels are working correctly.

Several connections may be made, depending on the condition of the lymphatic vessels. They are performed using a small cut just below the skin's surface. The surgery can be performed under local anaesthetic.

LVA protocols vary from centre to centre. At the ALERT Centre, we started performing LVA surgery in 2013. Our surgeons were trained by experts from Japan and supported by advanced imaging techniques introduced by A/Prof Hiroo Suami.

What management is required after LVA?

There are varied opinions on what garments, if any, you need after LVA surgery. Usually, your existing compression garment is fitted immediately after surgery and elevation of the limb is recommended for the first 24 hours. You can generally resume normal activities three to four days after surgery, then lifting, driving and gentle exercise after two weeks.

Apart from your compression garment, you should avoid direct pressure on the surgical site and high-intensity use of your arm (such as aerobic exercises or strength training) for at least one month after surgery.

You are also encouraged to continue with your usual conservative treatment by your lymphoedema therapist. This includes compression, massage, exercise and skin care, as discussed in **Chapter 6**, Complex Lymphoedema Therapy.

What are the success rates of LVA for lymphoedema?

Research on LVA mainly involves case studies from different major centres. These studies vary in terms of patient selection, surgical approach and postoperative protocols. A recent meta-analysis of LVA trials, encompassing nearly 6,500 patients, found a modest 35% reduction in excess arm circumference and 32% reduction in excess arm volume after microsurgery, with a decrease in the number of episodes of cellulitis (Meuli, 2023). Some patients I speak to say that their arm feels better or softer, even though they don't have any noticeable reduction in swelling.

In 2024, Koshima (the plastic surgeon who pioneered this technique) and his team published a comparison of 81 breast cancer patients with lymphoedema, treated either with conservative treatment (compression only, 52 patients) or surgical treatment (LVA plus compression, 29 patients). The study found that the surgical group had more sustained reductions in swelling and no further cases (0%) of cellulitis. In the conservative group, there was less reduction of swelling and the incidence of cellulitis increased to 15% (Shimbo, 2024). These results are promising but longer follow-up is required.

An important study from the Memorial Sloan Kettering Cancer Center in New York is investigating the use of immediate LVA – referred to as "immediate lymphatic reconstruction" (ILR) in the study – to prevent lymphoedema after breast cancer treatment. Patients undergoing axillary lymph node dissection were randomly allocated to either have ILR performed during their surgery, or have the regular surgery without it. So far there have been 72 patients in each group; the study will continue until all patients have been monitored for two years. However, results so far show that patients in the ILR group have a lower chance of developing lymphoedema (9.5% compared to 32% in the control group), better lymphatic function and better quality of life (Coriddi, 2023). More follow-up is required, but this treatment may become a standard of care in the future.

A similar, but non-randomised, study from the Harvard Medical School measured the incidence of lymphoedema in patients who had an ILR in addition to axillary dissection and radiation. In this study, 90 of 186 patients underwent successful ILR during their surgery, and the majority of patients went on to have radiation as well. The rate of chronic lymphoedema at the end of four years was only 9% (Granoff, 2023).

By contrast, a prospective comparison study following patients for four years did not find any difference between the group that had ILR with their axillary dissection and the group that did not (Levy, 2023). In this study, the term used was "lymphatic microsurgical preventive healing approach" (LYMPHA), but the procedure was the same, i.e. connecting lymphatic vessels to veins during surgery with the aim of preventing lymphoedema. Approximately one-third of patients in each group developed lymphoedema, suggesting that LYMPHA may not significantly reduce the long-term risk. Further research is needed to clarify the long-term benefits of this approach.

A meta-analysis by Johnson (2019) examined over 3,000 patients from 19 studies who received various combinations of axillary treatment with or without LYMPHA. The incidence of lymphoedema for patients receiving axillary lymph node dissection (ALND) alone was 14.1%, while ALND combined with regional lymph node radiation had a higher incidence of 33.4%. When ALND was performed with LYMPHA, lymphoedema rates dropped to 2.1%. Similarly, ALND combined with both radiation and LYMPHA showed a reduced incidence rate of 10.3%. These findings highlight that radiation to the lymph nodes increases the risk of lymphoedema, but integrating LYMPHA for patients having an axillary dissection significantly lowers their lymphoedema risk, whether or not they get radiation as well.

The authors followed up with another review of a much smaller group of patients – 97 patients who underwent axillary surgery with attempted ILR, as well as radiation in most cases (88%). The overall lymphoedema rate was 3.1%, and the findings supported lymphatic reconstruction during axillary surgery as a promising approach to prevent lymphoedema (Johnson, 2021). However, I would still advise that this technique remains experimental and we must await updated data to ensure these promising results are sustainable over time.

LYMPH NODE TRANSFER

Lymph node transfer (LNT) is probably the most complicated option for managing early lymphoedema. It is generally only offered to patients with early-stage lymphoedema who are not eligible for LVA due to the lack of potential join sites.

How does LNT work?

LNT involves transferring healthy lymph nodes from an unaffected part of the body to an area affected by lymphoedema. The goal of this surgery is that, over time, your body will incorporate the new nodes and they will begin to function and drain lymphatic fluid. This will improve your lymphatic circulation and potentially reduce the length of time you will need to wear compression garments.

The operation takes five to eight hours, as the procedure has two parts. The first is "harvesting" lymph nodes from another part of your body, called the donor site. Various locations have been used as donor sites, including the groin (inguinal nodes), the armpit (axillary nodes), under the jaw (submental nodes), around the colon (omental flap nodes) and above the collarbone (supraclavicular nodes).

A portion of tissue containing the lymph nodes, plus the surrounding fat, blood vessels and skin, is surgically removed from the donor site. The second part of the procedure involves moving this tissue to the area with lymphoedema, such as your armpit or wrist, and reconnecting the blood and lymphatic vessels.

What management is required after LNT?

The first two weeks after LNT are important for healing the surgical sites. You must keep pressure off the transferred lymph node tissue for this period. In most instances, this would be in the armpit, but it may be above or below the elbow or just above your wrist.

No direct manual pressure should be applied to the transferred tissue for one month after surgery. Your surgeon or lymphoedema therapist will guide you on when to reintroduce compression garments, typically around four to six weeks after surgery. After this period you can also go back to having manual lymphatic drainage on the affected limb.

What are the success rates of LNT for lymphoedema?

As with most research on lymphatic surgery, the success rates found in studies involving LNT are variable. It is essential to find a multidisciplinary team with experience in lymphatic imaging and surgery, who prefer to try all the conservative therapy approaches first. Ask your surgeon how many lymphatic microsurgery operations they have done and their rates of success and complications (Ngo, 2020).

One study reported complications such as chronic donor-site lymphoedema when the lymph nodes were harvested from the groin region, and found that LNT did not have any effect on volume reduction in the original site of lymphoedema (Vignes, 2013).

Another trial focused on evaluating the effectiveness of LNT compared to non-surgical approaches (Dionyssiou, 2016). Over three years, 83 female patients with stage 2 lymphoedema were examined. Among them, 36 cases were selected for the study and randomly divided into two groups: one group undergoing LNT followed by physiotherapy and compression, and the other managed solely with physiotherapy and compression. After a year of observation, significant findings emerged. Both groups experienced reduced limb volume, but those who underwent LNT saw a much greater volume reduction (57%) than the group without surgery (18%). Additionally, instances of infection were markedly lower in the LNT group, and patients reported improvements in pain, heaviness, and overall limb function.

Matilda's Story

In May 2019, I underwent a lumpectomy and lymph node clearance for carcinoma in my left breast. During Taxol chemotherapy, I first noticed swelling in the back of my hand and lower arm.

As a nurse and practice manager, I understood the implications and pursued all conservative treatments, including manual lymphatic drainage, compression garments, pneumatic compression, laser therapy, and taping. Despite wearing compression garments 24/7 and dedicating significant time daily, the swelling persisted, leaving me disheartened.

By August 2020, my left arm and hand were increasingly swollen and aching. I was referred to the ALERT Centre for indocyanine green (ICG) lymphatic mapping, which showed congestion in my hand and dysfunctional lymphatic vessels in my forearm.

In November 2020, with a noticeable size difference between my arms, I chose to proceed with lymphatic surgery. Lymph nodes from my right lower neck were transferred to my left elbow, and a lymphovenous anastomosis (LVA) bypassed blocked lymphatic pathways.

After surgery, my lymphoedema improved steadily. My arm softened, and the swelling reduced significantly. I had two cellulitis episodes before surgery but none since. I no longer wear a compression garment daily, only during exercise or as needed. A recent lymphoscintigram confirmed the functioning transferred lymph node.

This journey has been challenging, but I'm grateful for the option of surgery. I still perform self-massage as needed, and my arm now responds quickly. Though lymphoedema remains, it is far less burdensome and intrusive in my daily life.

WHAT ARE THE POSSIBLE COMPLICATIONS OF LYMPHATIC MICROSURGERY?

Complications from LVA are not very common; the procedure is performed just below the skin's surface, where there is minimal potential for damage. Possible complications include infection, impaired wound healing, reactions to the general anaesthetic, and allergic reactions to the ICG dye.

LNT is a more invasive procedure. Complications from LNT include general surgical complications such as bruising, infection, and poor wound healing; you may have pain at the donor site and if there is damage to the adjacent nerves, this will result in a patch of numbness. There is also the risk of lymphoedema developing at the donor lymph node site, which is a rare but serious complication (Vignes, 2013; Scaglioni, 2018). Scaglioni (2018), in a review of 24 studies involving LNT, found that the rate of donor-site lymphoedema in the groin region was about 2%, and that it did not occur at all in cases with an omental (colon) or head and neck donor site.

If blood supply to the flap (transferred tissue) is not successful, this can cause the flap to fail, known as necrosis. In this case, you may need to have another operation to repair, replace or remove the flap. Other potential complications of LNT include excess lymph leaking from the skin (lymphorrhoea) at the donor site. An abdominal hernia has also been reported.

SHOULD I CONSIDER LYMPHATIC MICROSURGERY?

Microsurgery is a highly specialised field undergoing ongoing research. It is expensive, and you must be cautious before deciding whether to have this procedure and where to get it done. With LVA, there is a risk that the procedure won't work and could damage your normal lymphatic vessels. At this stage, it is not a viable solution for most patients with lymphoedema. With LNT, there is a chance that taking lymph nodes from elsewhere in the body could lead to lymphoedema developing in a new location.

12

LYMPHOEDEMA PRECAUTIONS– FACT VS FICTION

In this chapter, I will present some of the older research that has guided the medical advice about the "dos and don'ts" of daily life, both for people living with lymphoedema and those who are at risk of developing it. For the most recent recommendations, we now have the 2024 Lymphology Association of North America (LANA) guidelines; at the end of the chapter I will include a summary of this evidence, sorting the recommendations based on whether you already have lymphoedema or are at risk of developing lymphoedema.

There are several precautions that people have taken over the years to try to avoid getting lymphoedema, or to prevent their lymphoedema from getting worse. For example, patients would avoid even the slightest interference with their arm after breast cancer treatment, or believe they could never travel by plane again. A lot of these theories have since been disproven, so it's important to know the difference between fact and fiction when it comes to lymphoedema precautions.

With lymphoedema, the bottom line is that you must try to get on with life; learn to take control of it rather than letting it control you. If you develop lymphoedema, you will need to get to know your new body. Speak to your doctor or therapist about your actual risk of lymphoedema. For example, if you are not obese or overweight, you had one sentinel node removed and you had no chemotherapy or radiation, your risk will be very low, less than one in 20 (5%). If you are at higher risk, e.g. because you are overweight or had treatment with an axillary lymph node dissection, radiation to the surrounding nodes and chemotherapy using taxanes, your risk may be as high as 30%. See **Chapter 3**, Risk Factors for Lymphoedema.

A study from MGH tracked the arm measurements of participating women before and after their breast cancer treatment to monitor for lymphoedema; the women were also asked about the frequency of blood tests, injections and air travel. Interestingly, the study found these activities didn't directly increase the risk of lymphoedema (Ferguson, 2016). However, some important factors did emerge – these included being overweight before treatment, having lymph nodes removed during surgery, and receiving radiation to the regional lymph nodes. In both the MGH study and the PREVENT study (Koelmeyer, 2022), which was research we did at ALERT in collaboration with Vanderbilt University, no link was found between flying and the development of lymphoedema.

Does this research mean that you needn't take any precautions? I don't think so. It is important to use your common sense, but don't panic if you forget one of your regular precautions from time to time, or if something unexpected happens. Do you always need to wear a lymphoedema alert band and warn health professionals to protect your arm? No. However, in most non-emergency situations, it is sensible to ask your health professional to use your other arm; if you have had surgery to both sides (bilateral), ask them to use the side where fewer lymph nodes were removed.

DO I NEED TO AVOID INJECTIONS IN MY AFFECTED ARM?

The concern about having injections in an arm affected by lymphoedema is common. However, procedures such as blood tests or vaccinations are often necessary, and you may not be able to avoid your affected or at-risk side every time. The most important priority is your health and well-being, and a fear of lymphoedema should not prevent you from having necessary medical procedures.

The risk of developing lymphoedema due to a simple blood test is extremely low. Jakes (2015) reviewed the available research studying this issue for patients with breast cancer, and concluded that there was no solid evidence that having a blood test (venepuncture) can cause lymphoedema.

Whenever possible, blood tests should be performed using the arm on the opposite side to your breast or axillary surgery. However, many of my patients find that they have no available veins on the opposite side due to the number of blood tests and chemotherapy injections they have already undergone. If this is the case and you do not have lymphoedema, it is generally safer and easier to use the same side as your cancer for blood tests, rather than veins in your foot or other less conventional locations. If you have upcoming tests or chemotherapy planned, an access port into a large vein might be the most appropriate and convenient option.

Whenever you have a blood test, it must be done carefully and cleanly, as an unexpected infection (cellulitis) can damage your lymphatic vessels. If you notice any signs of warmth or redness around the entry point after a blood test, see your doctor immediately, as you may need antibiotics. This is extremely rare with a carefully taken blood test (**Figure 12.1**). I will discuss cellulitis in **Chapter 13**, Prevention and Treatment of Cellulitis.

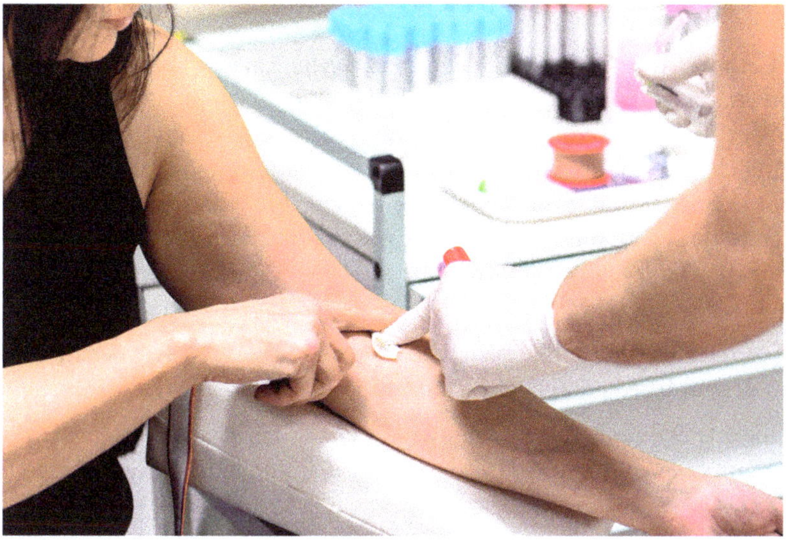

Figure 12.1

Blood tests should ideally be done on the opposite side to the breast or axilla where you had surgery. If that is not possible, you can use the affected side with care.

CAN I HAVE MY BLOOD PRESSURE TAKEN ON MY AFFECTED ARM?

Taking blood pressure on an arm affected by lymphoedema is generally safe. However, if you have existing lymphoedema, it's preferable to have your blood pressure taken on the other side. Although it's recommended to use the unaffected arm whenever possible, if this isn't an option or if your affected arm is used by mistake, don't stress – it's unlikely to cause harm. Manual blood pressure devices (**Figure 12.2**) are preferred over automatic ones, as taking blood pressure manually means the inflation of the cuff can be controlled, preventing excessive pressure from being applied to your arm.

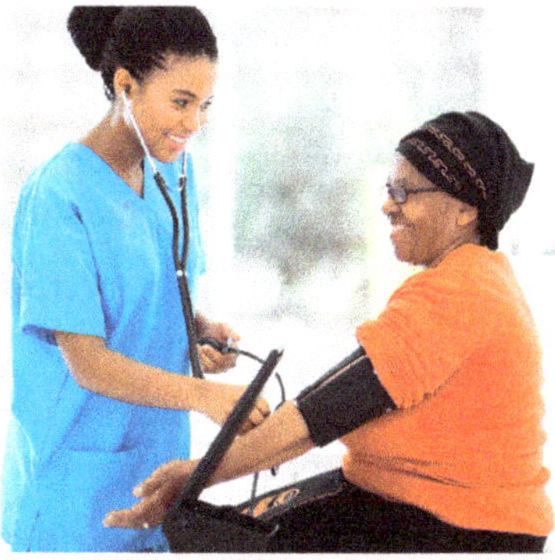

Figure 12.2

Having your blood pressure taken manually can be a way to avoid excessive pressure on your arm. However, there is no conclusive evidence to show that blood pressure measurement can trigger or exacerbate lymphoedema.

CAN I HAVE MEDICAL PROCEDURES ON MY AT-RISK ARM?

The short answer is "yes". Accidents can happen: you may need an operation on your arm after a fall, or need to have a skin cancer removed or treated with radiation. You may be in a situation where you have no good veins left after chemotherapy, and the only place to obtain a blood sample is from your at-risk arm. Use the other side if you can, but if you can't, procedures can be done with minimal risk, as long as they are clean and aseptic (free of germs). The risk of lymphoedema from a medical procedure is extremely low (Greene, 2015).

If you scratch your skin, wash it with an antiseptic wash such as Betadine, or an alcohol-based product like hand sanitiser, to reduce the risk of infection.

One rule of thumb is that if there have been two failed attempts at inserting a cannula in your arm, proceed to the at-risk side if there is good venous access (Jakes, 2015).

CAN I HAVE VACCINES IF I HAVE LYMPHOEDEMA?

For patients with established lymphoedema in one or more limbs, the British Lymphology Society (BLS) has developed guidelines about where to have your COVID-19 injection. This advice, of course, applies to other vaccines as well. In short, the BLS (2023) advises:

- If you have one arm affected by lymphoedema, both doses of the vaccine should be given in the unaffected, opposite arm.
- If you have had lymph nodes removed from one axilla, both doses of the vaccine should be given in the opposite arm.
- If both arms are affected by lymphoedema but not the legs, both doses of the vaccine should be given to the thighs or buttocks.
- If both arms and one leg are affected by lymphoedema, both doses of the vaccine should be given to the unaffected thigh or buttock.
- If both arms and legs are affected by lymphoedema, both doses of the vaccine should be given to the limb least affected by lymphoedema.

To read the BLS vaccination guidelines in full, visit https://www.thebls.com/documents-library/guidance-on-covid-19-and-flu-vaccinations-for-people-with-lymphoedema. (See also **Useful websites**, page 174.)

If you're on a blood thinner such as aspirin or warfarin, or you have a low **platelet count**, apply pressure to the vaccination site for about five minutes afterwards to prevent bruising.

For more information about vaccinations after a cancer diagnosis, see my book *Cancer & Vaccinations: Taking Control* (available via www.bcpublish.com).

WHEN CAN I EXERCISE AGAIN?

If you have lymphoedema, engaging in physical activity – including going to the gym – is encouraged. Exercise helps improve lymphatic flow and your overall well-being. In one of my recent studies (Boyages, 2022) we found that being overweight increased the risk of developing lymphoedema and that people with established lymphoedema gained more weight, so keeping fit with exercise is vital.

However, it's essential to start slowly and gradually increase the intensity. Consider consulting a personal trainer or exercise physiologist, as well as a lymphoedema therapist, to create a personalised exercise plan that suits your specific condition.

In 2011, a systematic review of 19 studies on exercise and its relationship to lymphoedema was conducted (Kwan, 2011). This review identified seven studies addressing resistance exercise, seven on aerobic and resistance exercise and five on other exercise modalities. The review concluded that slowly progressive exercise of varying modalities is not associated with the development or exacerbation of lymphoedema and can be safely pursued with proper supervision. Combined aerobic and resistance exercise appears safe, but more rigorous studies are needed (Kwan, 2011).

A study back in 2008 called the PAL (physical activity and lymphoedema) trial investigated the safety of progressive strength training in breast cancer survivors (Schmitz, 2009a, 2009b). This was a randomised clinical trial involving 295 women who had previously had breast cancer; approximately half (141 women) had existing lymphoedema, and the rest were at risk of developing lymphoedema. Participants who were randomly assigned to the treatment group attended exercise sessions twice a week for 12 months. The sessions included a cardiovascular warm-up, stretching and core exercises, followed by strength training using light weights that were gradually increased over the 12-month period. All participants wore a compression garment while exercising. The results showed that gradually progressive strength training (weightlifting) improved the participants' strength, physical function and quality of life, reduced their symptoms, without causing or exacerbating lymphoedema.

As a follow-up to the PAL trial, the same researchers conducted another study called the WISER (women in steady exercise research) trial, which looked at whether home-based exercise and weight-loss programs could be used to help overweight patients with breast cancer-related lymphoedema (Schmitz, 2019). Participants were randomised to different groups involving an exercise program, a weight-loss program or both, or to the control group (no intervention). However, this time the results showed that home-based interventions did not significantly improve lymphoedema outcomes. The authors recommended that a supervised, facility-based program of resistance exercise would be more beneficial for lymphoedema patients (Schmitz, 2019).

One Australian study randomised patients with existing lymphoedema into two groups, compression garment or no garment, and measured their L-Dex scores before and after moderate resistance exercise. The results showed that L-Dex scores decreased after exercise for the patients wearing a compression garment, but this was a temporary change; after 24 hours the L-Dex had gone back up again (Singh, 2015). However, the authors cautioned that most of their patients only had mild lymphoedema, so the results will not apply to everyone.

Given that wearing a compression garment does little harm and may do some good, my default advice would be that if you have been diagnosed with lymphoedema then you should wear your garment during exercise if possible. Some patients prefer to swim with their garment on. A wet garment cools the skin when the water evaporates, which is appreciated in countries with a hot climate.

CAN I GO BACK TO WEIGHTLIFTING?

One study by Schmitz (2010) found that weightlifting did not make lymphoedema worse. Breast cancer survivors from Philadelphia, who performed slowly progressive weightlifting twice a week for one year, were less likely to experience clinically significant increases in arm swelling than women in the control group.

The proportion of women who developed lymphoedema was 11% in the weightlifting group and 17% in the control group. Among women who had had five or more lymph nodes removed, the rate of developing lymphoedema was 7% in the weightlifting group and 22% in the control group, which was statistically significant (Schmitz, 2010).

DO EXTREME TEMPERATURES MAKE LYMPHOEDEMA WORSE?

A few studies such as Showalter (2013) showed that hot spas can increase the risk of lymphoedema. This is not certain, but if you're using a sauna or having a hot bath, there are some precautions you can take: don't overdo the heat, don't stay in for a long time, or simply hold your arm out of the spa. There is other evidence that heat does not increase the risk of lymphoedema, and may even improve it (Liu, 1993). In general, it's a good idea to follow the maxim of "everything in moderation".

CAN I GO TO THE BEACH?

Visiting the beach is safe for people with lymphoedema – just take normal precautions regarding sun exposure like everyone else. Use lots of sunscreen. Protecting yourself from the sun will prevent sunburn and minimise the risk of aggravating your lymphoedema symptoms, which may already be slightly worse in hotter months. A bad sunburn can also increase the risk of cellulitis, worsening your lymphoedema.

DO I NEED TO STOP GARDENING?

Gardening offers a dual benefit of physical activity and mental well-being, whether you are nurturing indoor plants or tending to an outdoor garden. Despite concerns about gardening for those with lymphoedema, if you take some common-sense precautions the risks of causing harm are very low.

Engaging with nature through gardening promotes a positive mindset and aids in stress reduction and relaxation, as evidenced by a 2017 meta-analysis highlighting its impact on overall quality of life and psychological health (Soga, 2017).

However, handling plants and bushes can lead to cuts and scrapes, which may introduce bacteria and exacerbate swelling. Similarly, insect bites pose a tiny risk of infection. The sharp tools used in gardening demand careful handling to avoid injuries, so it's important that you wear protective gloves. Over-exposure to the sun is another concern. Proper precautions such as sun protection (hat, sunscreen, SPF-protective clothing, etc.) and hydration are essential to reduce the risk of overheating your body or developing sunburn that can exacerbate your lymphoedema.

Ensure you moisturise daily to prevent cracked skin, which can become an entry point for infection. Wear long sleeves and gloves when gardening if possible (**Figure 12.3**). Avoid gardening outside in the middle of the day when the sun's rays are strongest, and always wear a hat. Spray some insect repellent on your clothing once you are outdoors, but always read the label on pest-control products.

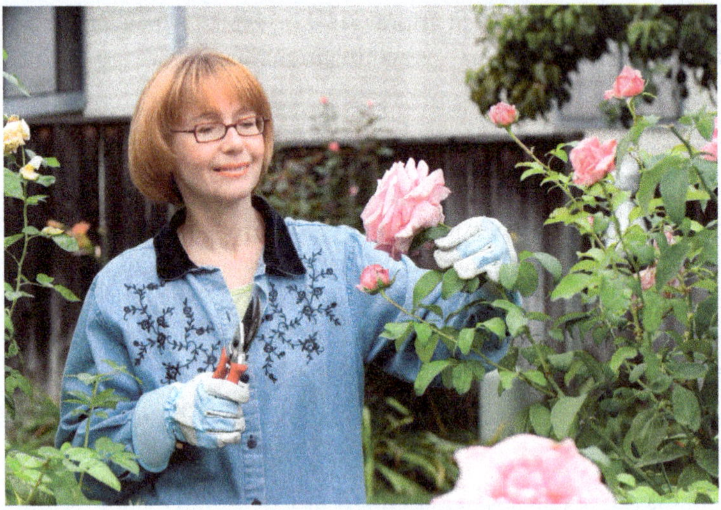

Figure 12.3

Get back to gardening as soon as you can, if it's something you enjoy, taking some common-sense precautions.

If you do injure yourself while gardening, clean the area thoroughly with soap and water, apply some hand sanitiser and consider using some antibacterial cream. These steps will help prevent infection. If the injury is more than a scratch, cover the wound with dry gauze or a bandage and see your doctor, particularly if the injury site is becoming warm, red and painful. Prompt attention to cuts, scrapes and bites can prevent complications like cellulitis.

It's a good idea to ask your doctor for a prescription for antibiotics to have on hand, so that if you see redness starting to spread in your swollen limb, you can fill the prescription and start taking them immediately. (However, you should still make an appointment to see your doctor.) Having some antihistamines at home is also a good idea in case you develop an allergic reaction to a plant scratch or an insect bite. If you have a localised itchy rash on your at-risk limb that doesn't settle down, try some hydrocortisone cream. If the rash gets worse, see your doctor urgently (see **Chapter 13**, Prevention and Treatment of Cellulitis).

All the above tips apply to people without lymphoedema as well. My advice is to take the above precautions and continue to enjoy your time in the garden.

CAN I TRAVEL IN A PLANE?

It is extremely unlikely that air travel can cause lymphoedema – the risk is low, even on high-altitude, long-haul flights. In my 40-year career, I have seen two patients who developed mild arm lymphoedema after flying long distances; however, it's also possible that they had subclinical lymphoedema which was undetected before the flight.

One study used bioimpedance spectroscopy to monitor women with previous breast cancer treatment who travelled to Queensland for a dragon boat regatta – 60 women flew from Canada and 12 from within Australia (Kilbreath, 2010). The women's arms were measured up to two weeks before their flight and on their arrival to Queensland. Forty of the women travelling from Canada were measured again six weeks after their return home.

The study reported four new cases of lymphoedema. Of the 42 patients who had travelled from Canada and had a prior axillary dissection, two women (5%) developed persistent lymphoedema. Lymphoedema did not develop in any patients who had been treated with a sentinel node biopsy; the authors rightly cautioned that this group of patients may have been fitter than others, so these results may not apply to the general population. Other researchers such as Ferguson (2016) and Koelmeyer (2022) have also found that air travel is not a significant risk factor for lymphoedema.

So, what does this mean in practice? Firstly, it is extremely rare for flying to cause lymphoedema, or to make your existing lymphoedema worse, if you have only had a sentinel node biopsy. Secondly, even after an axillary dissection it is not at all common.

RECOMMENDATION BY CATEGORY		
	People at risk of lymphoedema	People with confirmed lymphoedema
Air travel	No direct evidence linking air travel to lymphoedema; Consider garment if high-risk.	Wear your compression garments during flights.
Blood draws and injections	Isolated instances do not increase lymphoedema risk, but avoid if possible.	Avoid in the affected arm.
Blood pressure	Isolated BP measurements do not trigger lymphoedema.	Avoid blood pressure measurement in the affected arm.
Exercise	Supervised, slowly progressive resistance and aerobic exercise is safe and encouraged.	Supervised, slowly progressive resistance and aerobic exercise is safe and encouraged.
Heat/ temperature	Hot climate does not increase risk of lymphoedema. Avoid saunas.	Exposure to hot temperatures may increase swelling. Self-monitor and avoid saunas.
Surgical procedures	Discuss surgery risks with your surgeon and request lymphoedema checks before and after surgery.	Discuss surgery risks with your surgeon and request lymphoedema checks before and after surgery.
Skin care and infection	Protect skin with sunscreen and repellent. Seek urgent medical help if signs of infection.	Protect skin with sunscreen and repellent. Seek urgent medical help if signs of infection.

Table 12.1

Summary of the Lymphology Association of North America (LANA) risk reduction recommendations for breast cancer-related lymphoedema (Brunelle, 2024b).

Should I wear a compression garment on the plane?

This may seem obvious, but the first thing to note is that if you have a confirmed diagnosis of lymphoedema and already wear compression garments to manage your swelling, you should keep your garment on when you travel.

Some patients who are concerned about the risk of developing lymphoedema believe they should wear a garment during the flight as a preventative measure. In my practice, I tend to advise these patients that a compression garment is not necessary for relatively short flights (up to four to six hours' duration), such as domestic flights within Australia. For short flights without a garment, you can perform some self-massage during the flight and move your at-risk limb regularly to promote circulation.

If you a taking a longer flight of up to 14–24 hours, and if you are at risk of lymphoedema (see **Chapter 3**, Risk Factors for Lymphoedema), then I would advise a correctly fitted ready-to-wear compression sleeve as a precaution until more evidence becomes available. Wash and wear the sleeve before your flight to ensure it fits comfortably.

Many doctors would not go to these extremes given the mixed evidence on air travel, but it may help you to feel more at ease about travelling. Ultimately, we want you to get back to a normal life after cancer treatment, and not feel weighed down by unnecessary fears caused by outdated and unsubstantiated lymphoedema guidelines.

Discuss with your therapist and your doctor about travel tips and flight health; keep moving during your flight whenever possible, stay hydrated, and follow the in-flight instructions about moving and stretching your feet and legs to promote circulation. The main thing to know is that having cancer does not mean you are unable to travel.

LYMPHOEDEMA PRECAUTIONS – THE LATEST EVIDENCE

There are a lot of myths surrounding lymphoedema prevention; we have disproved some of these in this chapter already. Most of the "dos and don'ts" you hear about are not supported by strong evidence. For example, having an alert band labelling your arm as having lymphoedema is not required. If someone needs to take blood or put an **intravenous** (IV) cannula into that arm because of a medical emergency or an honest miscommunication, don't panic – just keep an eye on the area and monitor for redness or other signs of infection. (I will discuss infection in more detail in **Chapter 13**, Prevention and Treatment of Cellulitis.)

For up-to-date information about lymphoedema, including advice that is based on recent evidence, refer to professional organisations such as the Australasian Lymphology Association (https://www.lymphoedema.org.au), the British Lymphology Society (https://www.thebls.com) and the Lymphology Association of North America, or LANA (https://www.clt-lana.org). The latest recommendations at the time of writing are the 2024 risk reduction guidelines from LANA, published in October (Brunelle, 2024b). These guidelines relate to people who either have or are at risk of lymphoedema; an extract is shared in **Table 12.1**.

As you can see, these recommendations from LANA are quite practical and take a common-sense approach. As you adjust to life after cancer treatment and get used to your new body, try to get back to a lifestyle that is as close as possible to what you enjoyed before. It's normal to feel anxious about the risk of developing lymphoedema – or, if you have lymphoedema already, of making it worse – but it's important not to let this fear stop you from living your life. As you establish new routines you will find what works for you, and often you'll be able to take a trial-and-error approach. Above all, talk to your lymphoedema therapist: they are an excellent source of guidance and support, and can help you to manage existing lymphoedema or monitor closely for its onset.

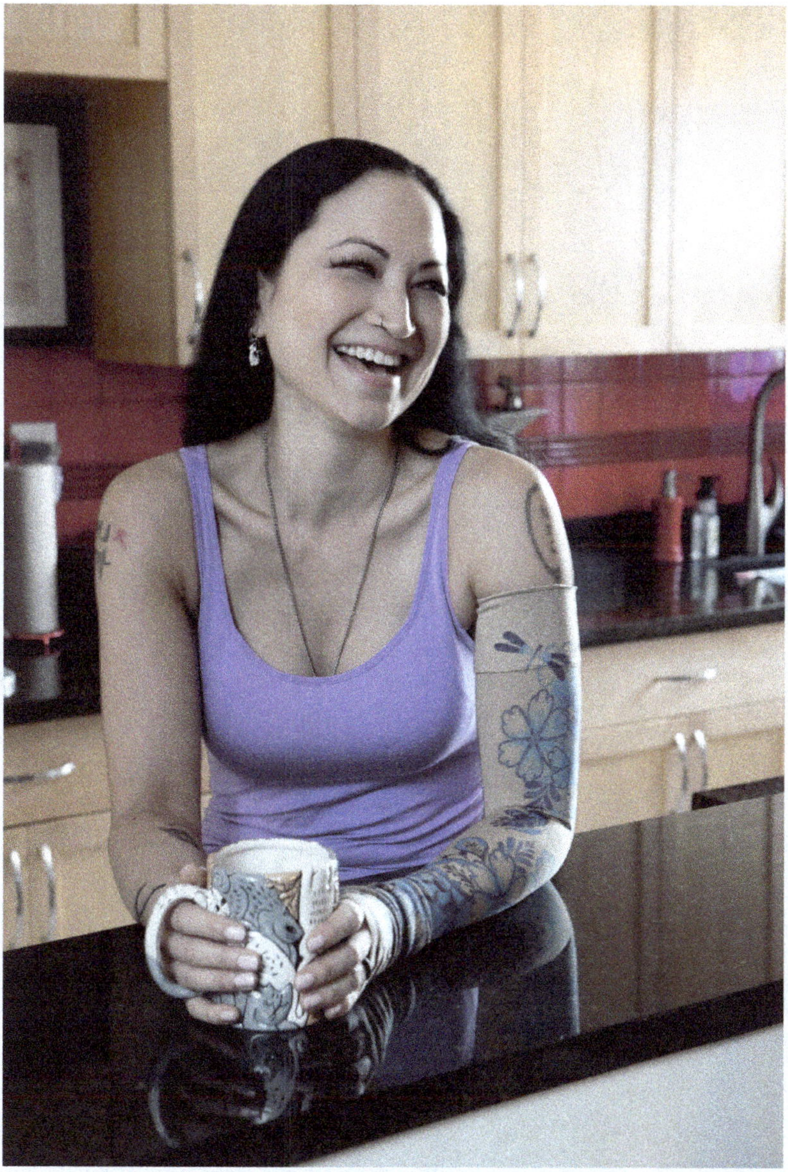

Figure 12.4

Try not to let lymphoedema get in the way of enjoying your life.
Copyright LympheDIVAs LLC, with permission.

13

PREVENTION AND TREATMENT OF CELLULITIS

WHAT IS CELLULITIS?

Cellulitis is a bacterial infection of the skin and underlying (subcutaneous) tissues. It presents with expanding redness, warmth, tenderness and swelling (**Figure 13.1**).

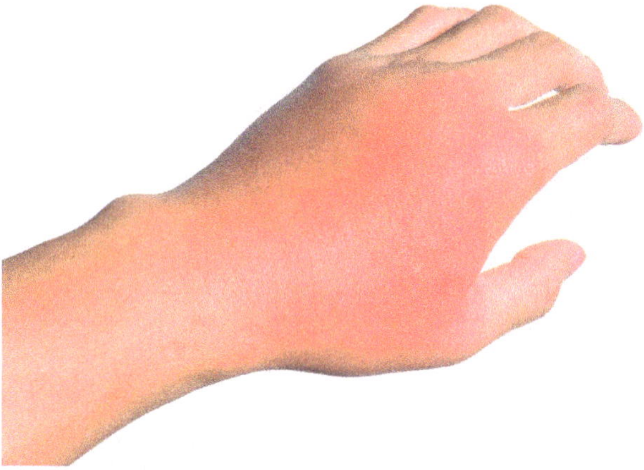

Figure 13.1

Redness with indistinct edges, warmth, swelling and tenderness are typical of cellulitis.

Risk factors for cellulitis include lymphoedema, previous episodes of cellulitis, obesity, pre-existing skin infections such as tinea, and possibly diabetes (Quirke, 2017). A large French study found a variety of risk factors for cellulitis in lymphoedema patients, depending on patient characteristics and lymphoedema type. For secondary upper limb lymphoedema, previous radiation treatment and younger age were associated with cellulitis (Vignes, 2022).

Cellulitis is similar to other infections called **erysipelas** and lymphangitis; while not exactly the same, these conditions are closely related, and the terms are often used interchangeably (Karlsson, 2022). Lymphangitis is inflammation of the lymphatic vessels, and often occurs at the same time as cellulitis. When the lymphatic vessels are inflamed, they appear as red streaky lines on the skin.

Lymphoedema of the breast, commonly known as breast oedema, can also become infected with cellulitis (see **Figure 13.2**). Cellulitis can also occur after recent surgery.

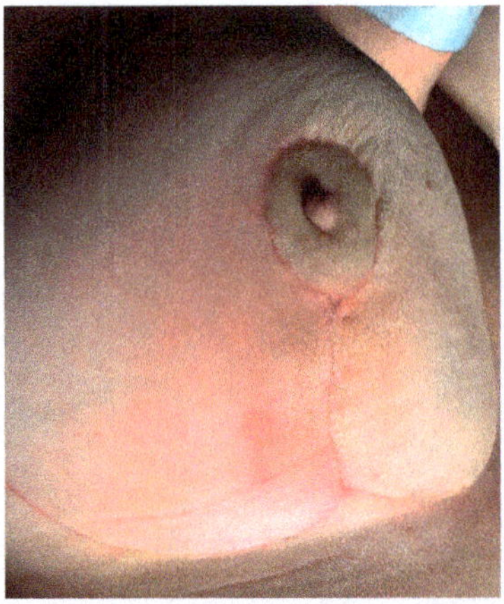

Figure 13.2

Cellulitis of the breast: redness with indistinct edges, warmth, swelling and tenderness surrounding the scars after recent surgery.

Sometimes skin affected by lymphoedema can be slightly pink, but not necessarily hot. It is like a faint blush and is called "lymphoedema rubra" (rubra means red in Latin). Lymphoedema rubra can be caused by inflammation or dilatation of the small blood vessels (capillaries) under your skin. If you press on the redness, it momentarily blanches (goes pale) around your finger. Lymphoedema rubra is often mistaken for cellulitis, but when antibiotics are prescribed they have no effect.

HOW COMMON IS CELLULITIS?

Cellulitis is a global health burden, responsible for more than 650,000 hospital admissions per year in the United States alone, and it can be lethal. It is a significant complication of breast cancer treatment.

Because the lymphatic vessels are part of the immune system and deliver bacteria to the lymph nodes for destruction, limbs affected by lymphoedema are immunocompromised, making them susceptible to bacterial infection and less able to fight off the bacteria.

In a study of 1,062 women who developed upper limb lymphoedema after breast cancer treatment, four in 10 women (39.5%) reported getting cellulitis. For half of these women, their cellulitis was recurrent, meaning it came back more than once. The risk of cellulitis was similar for patients with lymphoedema of the lower limb (Vignes, 2022).

In a study I led at Macquarie University, in partnership with the Breast Cancer Network Australia and the Australasian Lymphology Association, we conducted a national survey of 361 women who had breast cancer with lymphoedema (152 women) and breast cancer without lymphoedema (209 women).

Twenty-five patients (16%) reported having an episode of cellulitis in the past year. The incidence of cellulitis was 8% in patients with subclinical or mild lymphoedema, and 30% in patients with more extensive lymphoedema. This is a significant concern, as it means nearly one in three women with moderate or severe lymphoedema had experienced cellulitis within the last year (Boyages, 2017).

HOW DO I KNOW IF I HAVE CELLULITIS?

Cellulitis can present as a "local" problem, meaning it only affects a certain part of the body, or it can be "systemic", causing symptoms that affect your whole body (Raff, 2016).

Local effects

Local effects can be seen or felt in the affected area, such as your hand, arm or leg. Cellulitis can occur anywhere, but most often affects the limbs.

- Mild to moderate: Pain, swelling, redness and warmth
- Severe: Blisters, pustules or abscess formation.

Systemic effects

The systemic effects of cellulitis can be seen or felt in the whole body, causing changes in your vital signs (Raff, 2016). For example:

- Moderate:
    - Temperature >38°C (100.4°F)
    - Heart rate >90 beats per minute
    - Respiratory rate >20 breaths per minute
    - White blood cell count >12,000 or <4,000 per mm^3
    - Low blood pressure, e.g. systolic (the top number) <90 mmHg

- Severe:
    - More than two of the above systemic effects *and*
    - Low blood pressure *or*
    - Rapid disease progression.

WHAT SHOULD I DO IF I THINK I HAVE CELLULITIS?

Seek medical advice as soon as possible, on the same day you notice any symptoms. Cellulitis can progress very quickly, and stopping it in its tracks is essential. Act quickly and you can avoid an admission to hospital.

If you are prone to recurrent episodes of cellulitis, you should always have a supply of antibiotics, or at least a prescription, ready at home. Bring a course of antibiotics with you when you travel and start taking them when you see the first sign of redness. It is also helpful to mark out the outline of your rash with a marker pen when you first develop cellulitis. This allows you to see if the rash is spreading.

Your medical team may do some blood tests if you have some of the systemic effects mentioned above, or if your cellulitis is extensive and expanding quickly. However, if cellulitis is suspected, you should not wait for the test results to start antibiotics.

Blood tests will include:

- A full blood count (FBC) to see if your white blood cells are too high or too low, which could indicate that your immune system is fighting an infection.
- Erythrocyte sedimentation rate (ESR), also called the "sed rate", which detects inflammation in the body. This test measures how quickly red blood cells settle to the bottom of a test tube: the faster the cells settle within an hour, the higher the chance that your cellulitis is causing systemic effects.
- A C-reactive protein (CRP) test, which is another way to check for infection or inflammation. CRP is a protein found in the blood, and its levels increase when there is inflammation in the body.
- If you have any pustules or areas of broken skin, a swab will be taken to test for bacteria and identify which antibiotics will

work for you. Some bacteria, such as methicillin-resistant Staphylococcus aureus (MRSA), are antibiotic-resistant. These bugs are resistant to standard antibiotic therapy, so different treatment combinations are required.

HOW IS CELLULITIS TREATED?

Cellulitis is a bacterial infection, so the main treatment is antibiotics. Antibiotics are usually given as a tablet or capsule (orally). You may need to have antibiotics in hospital via a drip (intravenously) if your infection is severe.

When it comes to the prescribing the right antibiotic, there is no correct answer. I usually prescribe oral cephalexin, 500mg every six hours.

The British Lymphology Society (BLS) has developed comprehensive guidelines on the management of cellulitis, including antibiotic use. They advise oral flucloxacillin, 500–1000mg every six hours (with preference for the lower dose), arguing that this drug works best against streptococcus and staphylococcus bacteria, the common culprits that cause cellulitis (BLS, 2022). You can find the guidelines on the BLS website: visit https://www.thebls.com/documents-library/guidelines-on-the-management-of-cellulitis-in-lymphoedema (or see **Useful websites**, page 174).

A review from Harvard Medical School (Raff, 2016) advises:

- Cephalexin *or*
- Dicloxacillin *or*
- Phenoxymethylpenicillin ("Penicillin V") *or*
- Amoxicillin/clavulanate.

If there is a true penicillin allergy, consider:

- Clindamycin *or*
- Clarithromycin (if you can take a "macrolide" antibiotic) *or*
- Doxycycline (if you cannot take a macrolide, e.g. because you're on a statin medication).

If there are more than two systemic (whole-body) effects, intravenous (IV) antibiotics given via a drip are recommended. The BLS advises switching to clindamycin (300mg every six hours) or cephalexin if the first-line antibiotic doesn't work.

The Australasian Lymphology Association (ALA) last updated its guidelines in 2015. To read the ALA consensus guideline on the management of cellulitis in lymphoedema, visit https://www.lymphoedema.org.au/about-lymphoedema/consensus-guideline/ (or see **Useful websites**, page 174).

How long should I take antibiotics for?

Although many general antibiotic guidelines advise only five to seven days of antibiotic treatment, the BLS recommends a full 14-day course of antibiotics for cellulitis in lymphoedema. They note that shorter courses of antibiotics often lead to early recurrence of cellulitis, implying an incomplete resolution of the infection.

In addition, I usually suggest eating yoghurt or taking probiotics to help restore your normal gut flora, which can be affected by antibiotics. Disruption of the microorganisms in your gut can lead to overgrowth of a dangerous bacteria called Clostridium difficile (*C. diff*), which causes severe diarrhoea.

During periods of acute infection, the level of arm or leg compression should be reduced or removed if it is too painful, and any form of lymphatic massage should be discontinued. You can go back to wearing your compression garment once it is comfortable to do so, as cellulitis generally increases the amount of swelling and the garment can be beneficial.

CAN CELLULITIS BE PREVENTED?

If you are having surgery on your arm, it's a good idea to have a prophylactic course of antibiotics starting one day before surgery and continuing for five to seven days after surgery. Types of surgery that you may have on your arm include skin cancer removal, carpal tunnel surgery and lymphoedema surgery (see **Chapter 10**, Liposuction for Lymphoedema and **Chapter 11**, Lymphatic Microsurgery).

Antibiotic prophylaxis

Taking prophylactic antibiotics for long periods is not usually recommended. The BLS advises that antibiotic prophylaxis should only be considered in patients who have had two or more episodes of cellulitis in the previous year.

If any of the following questions are answered "yes" then your doctor should consider holding off on prescribing you prophylactic antibiotics:

- Was it possible that not all episodes were bacterial cellulitis?
- Were the episodes incompletely treated cellulitis that recurred quickly after a short course of antibiotics?
- Was there a clear reversible cause of infection (e.g. dermatitis) where treatment of the cause may prevent future attacks?

According to the BLS guidelines:

- If antibiotic prophylaxis is indicated, the first choice should be phenoxymethylpenicillin 250mg every 12 hours (or 500mg every 12 hours if BMI ≥33).
- For those allergic to penicillin, clarithromycin 250mg daily is recommended. Clarithromycin is known as a macrolide.
- For patients with a penicillin allergy who can't take macrolides, doxycycline 100mg daily is recommended.
- If the response to first-line prophylactic antibiotics is inadequate, alternative strategies such as cephalexin 125mg daily or clindamycin 150mg daily may need to be considered.

The review by Raff (2016) also advised that other antibiotics are appropriate for prophylaxis, including:

- Oral penicillin 250mg or 1g twice daily
- Erythromycin 250mg twice daily
- Dicloxacillin 500mg twice daily
- Clindamycin 150mg daily
- Intramuscular benzathine penicillin 1.2 million units/month, for durations as variable as one week to 12 months.

In a 2013 randomised controlled trial, 274 patients with recurrent cellulitis were given either prophylactic penicillin (250mg, twice daily) or a placebo for 12 months. Thirty of 136 patients (22%) in the penicillin group experienced a return of their cellulitis, compared to 51 of 138 patients (37%) in the placebo group. The results showed that antibiotic prophylaxis reduced the risk of recurrent leg cellulitis; however, this effect diminished when the penicillin was discontinued (Thomas, 2013).

It is recommended that after one year of successful prophylaxis, discontinuation of antibiotics should be considered; however, you may continue for an extra year if there are ongoing significant risk factors for cellulitis. If there are no further episodes of cellulitis during this period, antibiotic prophylaxis should be stopped (BLS, 2022).

Other prevention methods

There is evidence that good lymphoedema care using complex lymphoedema therapy (CLT) can help to prevent cellulitis. Skin care is vital, including daily moisturising to avoid cracks in the skin that may introduce infection. Make sure there are no signs of fungal infection at the base of your nails or between your fingers that may require antifungal cream. Cut your finger and toenails using clippers; cut toenails straight across to prevent ingrown nails, and push back the cuticles on your fingers rather than cutting them. It's also important to see a podiatrist from time to time. For more on skin care, see **Chapter** 7, Skin Care and Lymphoedema.

Will disinfecting my skin prevent cellulitis?

I once attended a wound care session at a lymphoedema conference where one of the speakers advised everyone to have a "brown bath" once a week. This involves splashing iodine solution (such as Betadine) all over your skin in the shower, leaving it there for a minute or so, and then washing it off with soap. It can make a bit of a mess!

The theory behind this is that iodine reduces the amount of bacteria on your skin, so there is less chance that cuts or cracks can lead to infection. Another wash you can use is chlorhexidine, an antiseptic readily available at your local chemist. After that conference, I became a "brown bath" convert; when I remember, I still do it once a week.

In researching this book, I decided to see if any science existed behind this doctor's recommendation. I found one randomised trial comparing different methods for removing Staphylococcus aureus ("staph") from the skin to reduce infection (Fritz, 2011).

Three hundred patients with skin or soft tissue infections and staph colonisation were given different treatments for five days:

- Daily body wash with 4% chlorhexidine solution, plus antibiotic ointment (mupirocin) in the nose
- Daily 15-minute soak in a diluted bleach bath (1/4 cup of 6% sodium hypochlorite per bathtub of water), plus mupirocin in the nose
- Education only (no treatment) for the control group.

Although the patients in both treatment groups had roughly the same chance of re-developing a skin infection after six months as the control group (see **Table 13.1**), the rate of infection was slightly lower in the chlorhexidine group. I would also assume that a weekly program would be more effective than using the treatment for only five days.

	RECURRENT SKIN/SOFT TISSUE INFECTION		
	After 1 month	after 4 months	after 6 months
TREATMENT TYPE			
Chlorhexidine wash	11%	33%	43%
Bleach bath	22%	35%	50%
No treatment	26%	41%	54%

Table 13.1

Rate of developing skin and soft tissue infection after treatment to eradicate *S. aureus* (staph) from the skin (Fritz, 2011).

My view is that this type of treatment probably does no harm, and options would include the iodine wash (such as Betadine), a chlorhexidine wash (such as Hibiclens), or the diluted bleach bath as a less expensive option.

Recently, I recommended the brown bath to one of my patients who was getting recurrent cellulitis. To my amusement, her lymphoedema therapist mentioned what she termed the "Boyages brown bath" in her report! I really can't take credit for this novel research.

Josie's Story

I was diagnosed with breast cancer in May 2008, and by December I had developed lymphoedema. As a cancer survivor, I am grateful for every day I wake up. The journey doesn't end with remission. One of the constant reminders of my experience is lymphoedema, a chronic condition I now live with. Every day, I wear a compression sleeve, a tangible symbol of my battle with cancer.

In 2009, an infection from a breast implant triggered cellulitis, landing me in the hospital. I had another bout of cellulitis in 2023, when I was hospitalised again. Over the years, I've undergone at least four extensive massage therapy sessions for lymphoedema and have even bought a pneumatic pump to try and keep it more under control.

One of the most helpful interventions has been ICG lymphatic mapping. This mapping, which I strongly recommend to patients at a moderate stage, has been invaluable in understanding my condition better. It provides a clear picture of the lymphatic pathways, helping to tailor treatments and manage the condition more effectively.

While there are provisions to claim expenses for various activities like gym classes, jogging, remedial massage, and swimming lessons, the support for managing lymphoedema falls short. I can claim only $50 per garment, yet each sleeve costs me $250.

Josie's Story cont'd

I need at least four of these a year to manage my condition effectively. This is not a one-time purchase but an ongoing expense for a chronic condition, not a lifestyle choice.

The wearing of the sleeve is more than a financial burden; it's an emotional one. It serves as a daily reminder of my cancer experience, something I literally "wear on my sleeve". While I strive to put the past behind me, the sleeve constantly reminds me that the journey continues.

Navigating life as a cancer survivor comes with its unique set of challenges. Each day, I balance gratitude for my survival with the reality of my ongoing medical needs. Though helpful, the existing support systems often don't fully address the chronic nature of conditions like lymphoedema. Despite these challenges, I continue to move forward, embracing each day with resilience and hope.

14

BREAST OEDEMA

WHAT IS BREAST OEDEMA?

Breast oedema is lymphoedema that occurs in the breast. While it shares a lot of similarities with the lymphoedema in the limbs that we've been discussing throughout this book, breast oedema comes with its own particular challenges. The risk of oedema can be higher in the breast due to radiation of both the breast tissue and the axillary lymph nodes. Breast oedema can also be more difficult to detect in the early stages.

The most common cause of breast oedema is surgery with or without radiation. It can also be seen after mastitis, trauma to the breast, and more rarely with problems of circulation such as heart failure. When breast oedema occurs at the time of breast cancer diagnosis, before any surgery or radiation has been performed, it may be a sign of an advanced type of cancer called **inflammatory breast cancer**. In this case, there will be multiple malignant lymph nodes blocking the lymphatic circulation in the axilla, or a blockage of the lymphatic system under the skin, which can sometimes be associated with redness of the breast. When redness is present, this may indicate advanced breast cancer.

In this chapter, I will not be discussing this type of malignant breast oedema. However, if you are a therapist reading this book, always keep this possibility in mind if breast oedema occurs unexpectedly, perhaps many years after treatment, or if it comes with associated symptoms of pain in the axilla or breast, nodularity in the axilla or skin thickening. If you are concerned about your clinical findings or worried that your therapy is not working, refer the patient to their medical team for an urgent opinion.

HOW COMMON IS BREAST OEDEMA?

The prevalence of breast oedema varies among individuals and is influenced by multiple factors. Studies have reported that breast oedema can occur in a significant proportion of breast cancer survivors, ranging from a low of 0% to a high of 90% (Verbelen, 2014; Brunelle, 2024a). This broad range is due to the fact that there are different ways of measuring and diagnosing breast oedema.

Radiation oncologist Daniel Clarke classified breast oedema in 74 patients treated with lumpectomy and radiation as follows:

- Mild – minor increase in breast size
- Moderate – obvious oedema with **peau d'orange** and patients complaining of heaviness
- Severe – caused significant symptoms such as pain or resulted in a poor cosmetic result.

Clarke was one of the first investigators to look at the extent of treatment to the axilla and incidence of breast oedema (Clarke, 1982). In 1988, I repeated his study in a group of 121 patients treated at Westmead Hospital (Boyages, 1988). **Table 14.1** shows the results of both studies:

	INCIDENCE OF BREAST OEDEMA	
	Axillary dissection	Axillary radiation
Stanford		
Any breast oedema	78%	3%
Westmead		
Any breast oedema	73%	16%
Moderate or severe breast oedema	13%	4%

Table 14.1

Comparison of results from studies by Clarke (1982) at Stanford and Boyages (1988) at Westmead on the incidence of breast oedema after different axillary treatments.

In both the Stanford and Westmead studies, the incidence of breast oedema was higher in the first 6–12 months after radiation. Breast oedema was particularly high when an axillary dissection was done and relatively low when radiation was given. These days, not many patients are given axillary radiation as their only treatment. Most would have some type of surgical intervention, such as a sentinel node biopsy.

Since the introduction of the sentinel node biopsy procedure, more patients have breast preservation rather than undergoing a mastectomy. This has increased the importance of monitoring the breast for lymphoedema.

One of the reasons for such a wide range in the incidence of breast oedema is that it depends on how and when breast oedema was measured.

The incidence rate may be very high when using a breast ultrasound to measure skin thickness, but would an ultrasound be done if the patient had no symptoms? Two excellent review papers (Verbelen, 2014; Boughey, 2014) summarised the issues as follows:

- There is a marked variation in breast oedema incidence due to different measurement techniques: patient surveys, various diagnostic tests or photos.
- Limited studies have measured breast oedema over time for the same group of patients.
- Like arm oedema, the average overall incidence is 20%, but only 5% for moderate or severe breast oedema.
- The incidence of breast oedema is higher when measured by ultra sound (70–90%), mammography (69%) or MRI (64%).
- Higher BMI and certain locations of the surgical incision (lower inner quadrant and upper outer quadrant) increase the incidence of breast oedema.

My own experience, supported by at least one good study (Rönkä, 2004), is that the incidence of breast oedema varies by the location (quadrant) of the original cancer in the breast and the extent of surgery to the axilla as follows:

- Low risk:
    - ¤ Upper quadrants and sentinel node biopsy
- Moderate risk:
    - ¤ Upper quadrants and axillary dissection
    - ¤ Lower quadrants and sentinel node biopsy
- High risk:
    - ¤ Lower quadrants and axillary dissection
    - ¤ Lower quadrants and axillary dissection plus radiation.

An important point here is that many of my patients don't even know they have breast oedema. Often it is only a small amount in the area around their scar, or the nipple area (areola) may be slightly thickened or lighter. Usually the oedema causes no problems if it is only minor.

HOW DOES BREAST OEDEMA AFFECT QUALITY OF LIFE?

I see many other patients who are affected by breast oedema. They suffer from heaviness, swelling, pain and sometimes recurring infections. As with arm lymphoedema, the condition is often a daily reminder of their previous cancer treatment, and they can become frustrated that clinicians are ignoring their problem or that therapies only give temporary relief. There is not a lot of research about the impact of breast oedema on a patient's feelings and daily life.

One study aimed to address the lack of research data on breast oedema, carefully studying 800 patients before radiation treatment and at various intervals up to 18 months after treatment (Young-Afat, 2019). A quarter of all patients (25%) reported breast oedema at some point. The highest rate of breast oedema occurred at six months post-radiation, affecting one in eight patients (12%).

Several factors were identified as determinants of breast oedema, including larger tumour size, oncoplastic surgery, axillary lymph node dissection, radiotherapy to the surrounding region, radiotherapy boost to the tumour bed, and adjuvant chemotherapy.

Importantly, breast oedema was independently associated with several negative impacts on quality of life. It was linked to increased breast pain, and patients experienced a decrease in well-being, impaired ability to perform daily tasks, and negative psychological consequences related to changes in their breast appearance.

HOW IS BREAST OEDEMA DIAGNOSED?

Clinical features

Diagnosing breast oedema involves recognising specific clinical features, including breast swelling, heaviness, tightness, and skin changes (such as thickening or indentation). Peau d'orange, meaning "skin of the orange" in French, is a condition characterised by small pits or indentations on the skin surface, where the affected area resembles the texture and appearance of an orange peel. This condition occurs due to the build-up of fluid and swelling in the underlying tissues, causing the skin to thicken and develop a pitted or pebbled texture (see **Figures 14.1–14.4**).

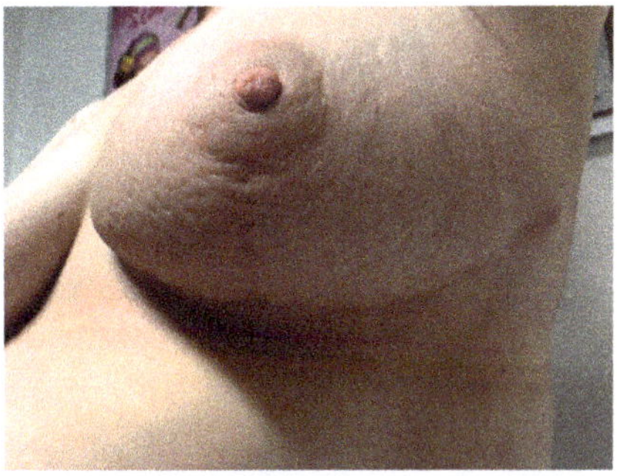

Figure 14.1

Left-sided breast oedema: notable indicators include swelling, tenderness, heaviness, skin thickening, indentations from a bra, areola thickening and skin dimpling (peau d'orange).

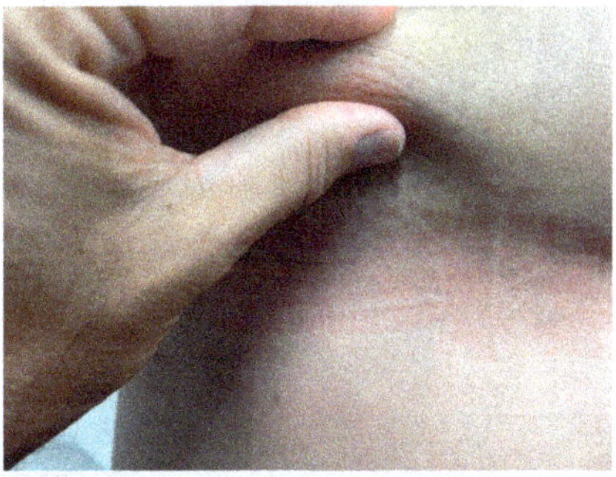

Figure 14.2

Gently squeezing the skin (with patient permission) allows the peau d'orange or dimpling to be more pronounced. I always shine the patient examination light at a tangent across the breast to highlight the dimpling.

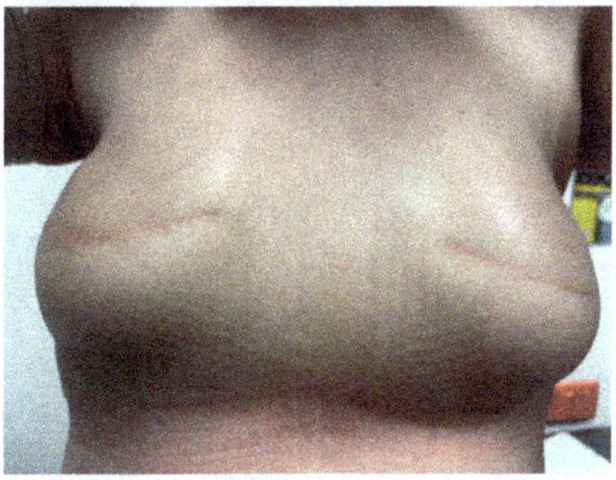

Figure 14.3

Oedema can also occur after a mastectomy on the skin of the chest wall. In this patient, you can see the dimpling and thickened skin, mainly under the mastectomy scars, which obstruct the flow of lymphatic fluid.

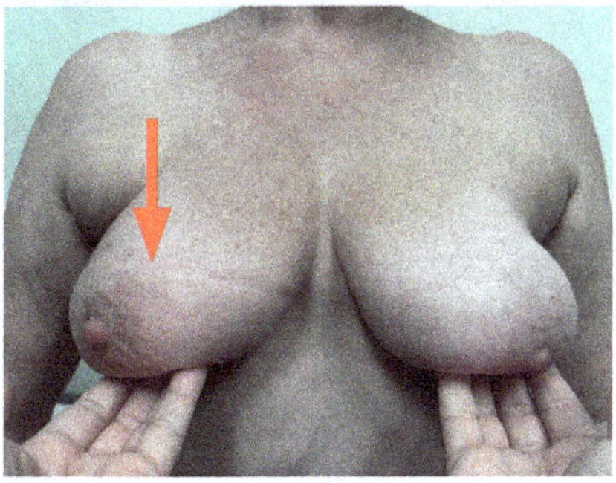

Figure 14.4

Lift your breasts up (or if you are a doctor or therapist, ask the patient's permission to lift both breasts), which will show an obvious difference in weight between the treated and untreated breast because of oedema. On the right breast, a bra has caused indentation in the skin above the nipple (arrowed).

Tissue dielectric constant

Measurement of tissue dielectric constant (TDC) involves scanning your affected breast with a non-invasive device called a moisture meter (**Figure 4.10**) and comparing the measurement to that of your unaffected breast. Typically, at least five measurements are taken (one in each breast quadrant and one around the nipple). The moisture meter converts the TDC to a percentage water content to show the amount of lymphatic fluid present in the skin of your breast. This simple technique can provide objective information about the severity of breast oedema and help to monitor your response to treatment (Johansson, 2016). For more information on moisture meters, see **Chapter 4**, Clinical Assessment and Tests.

Breast imaging

Mammography and breast ultrasound are routinely done after breast-conserving surgery and radiation to find the small number of patients who develop a new cancer in the affected breast or on the opposite side.

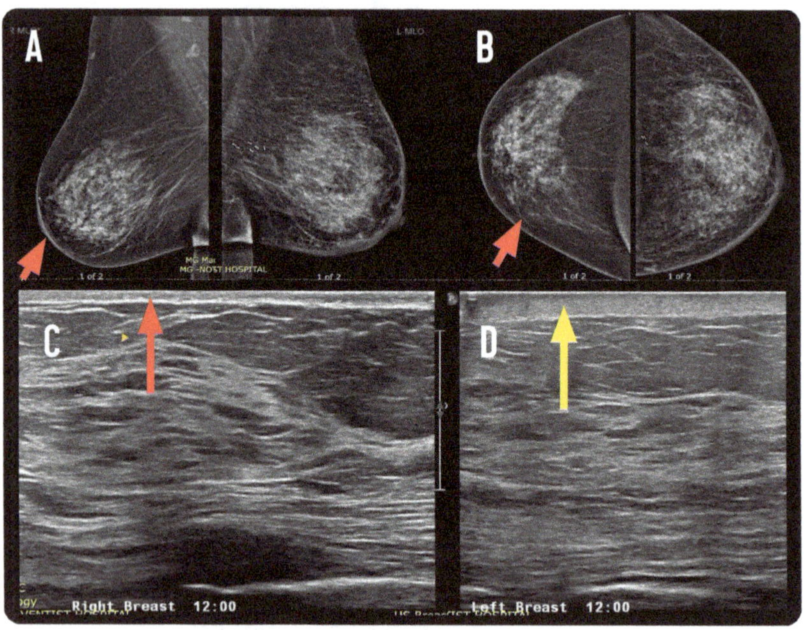

Figure 14.5

A: Mammogram (side view), B: mammogram (top view), C: breast ultrasound. The red arrows show normal skin on the right, and the yellow arrow shows thickened skin on the left.

When I see a patient who is worried about heaviness in her breast, I look at the breast imaging, preferably from before her surgery through to the latest images that are available. In **Figure 14.5**, the yellow arrow shows how the skin gets thicker on the mammogram or ultrasound on the treatment side compared the untreated side (red arrows). This is also seen in views of a breast ultrasound.

ICG lymphography

Indocyanine green (ICG) lymphography is a specialised imaging technique that involves injecting a fluorescent green dye into the breast tissue to assess lymphatic flow. I first mentioned it in **Chapter 4**, Clinical Assessment and Tests. In testing for breast oedema, we ask the patient to wear a gown with her clothes removed above the waist. The skin is cleaned and then numbed with a special applicator called a CoolSense device, which cools the skin.

A tiny amount (less than half a millilitre) of ICG dye is injected under the skin using a fine needle. Immediately following the injections, continuous scanning of lymphatic vessels with a near-infrared camera is performed. If ICG does not extend to the breast following injections in the upper abdomen, a further ICG injection is given in the breast itself.

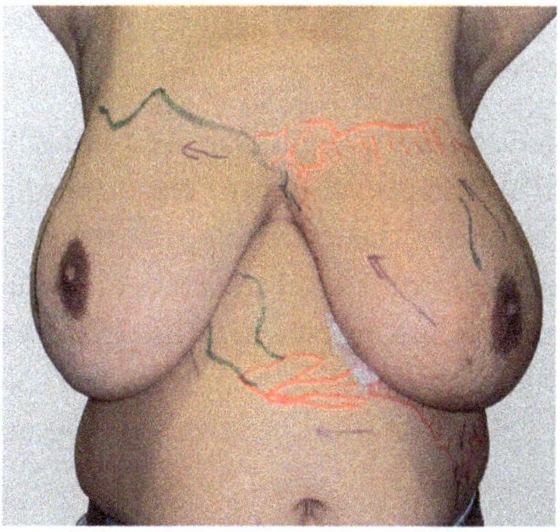

Figure 14.6

Marking on the skin done during ICG lymphography. New lymphatic pathways to the opposite armpit via nodes behind the breastbone and towards the left groin are shown in green. Collections of lymphatic fluid, called "dermal backflow", are shown in red.

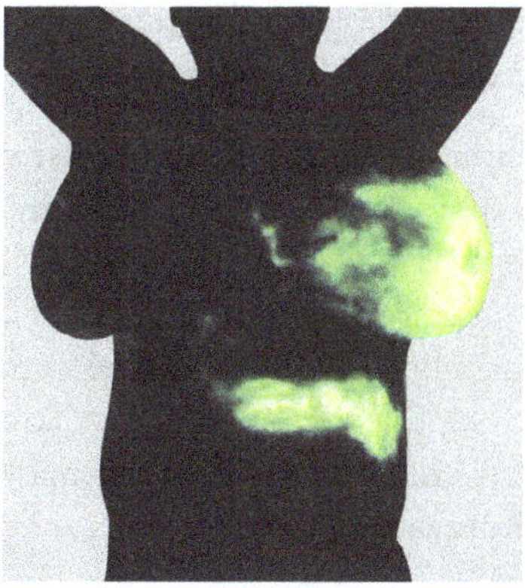

Figure 14.7

Marked collections of lymphatic fluid detected by an infrared camera using infrared dye. This is the same patient as in Figure 14.4.

Throughout the scanning procedure, felt pens are used to mark lymphatic vessels and areas of dermal backflow on the skin (**Figure 14.6**) based on the images on the computer monitor (**Figure 14.7**)

HOW IS BREAST OEDEMA TREATED?

Skin care

Proper skin care is essential in managing breast oedema, including keeping the skin clean, moisturised and protected to prevent infection and promote healing. Moisturise your treated breast every day after showering or bathing. (See also **Chapter 7**, Skin Care and Lymphoedema.)

Exercise

Regular exercise for the upper body and activities that move your body in different ways can improve your lymphatic circulation. This can help decrease swelling and improve how you feel overall.

In one randomised controlled trial conducted by Kilbreath (2020), women with stable breast oedema were randomised into an exercise group (41 women) or a control group (47 women). The exercise group completed a 12-week program that combined aerobic and resistance training, supervised weekly by an accredited exercise physiologist.

Physical changes in the breast were assessed using ultrasound imaging and bioimpedance spectroscopy (BIS). Patient symptoms were recorded using two validated quality-of-life surveys. The exercise group reported a greater reduction in breast-related symptoms than the control group, and a decrease in fluid level in the skin as measured with BIS. There was no significant difference in skin thickness detected by ultrasound. No exacerbations of lymphoedema were observed from the exercise program (Kilbreath, 2020).

Manual lymphatic drainage

Manual lymphatic drainage (MLD) is a specialised massage technique performed by trained lymphoedema therapists to stimulate lymphatic flow, aid fluid drainage and reduce swelling in the affected breast (see **Chapter 6**, Complex Lymphoedema Therapy). MLD is an important tool in managing your breast oedema.

Compression bra/vest

Wearing a compression bra or vest provides external support to the breast tissue, promotes lymphatic flow and helps reduce swelling. Proper fitting and guidance from a healthcare professional is crucial. A compression bra with a Mobiderm insert is a valuable tool to manage your breast oedema. In this innovative combination, the bra provides targeted compression and support to alleviate swelling, while the Mobiderm insert offers gentle massage and stimulation to promote lymphatic drainage and reduce fluid build-up (**Figure 14.8**). Together, they create a soothing and effective solution to help you find comfort and aid in healing. One of my patients, mentioned earlier in **Figure 14.6**, has had a marked improvement in her quality of life by wearing a firm compression bra daily. Her peau d'orange is hardly visible and her left breast is much less swollen, almost the same weight as the other side (see **Figure 14.9**).

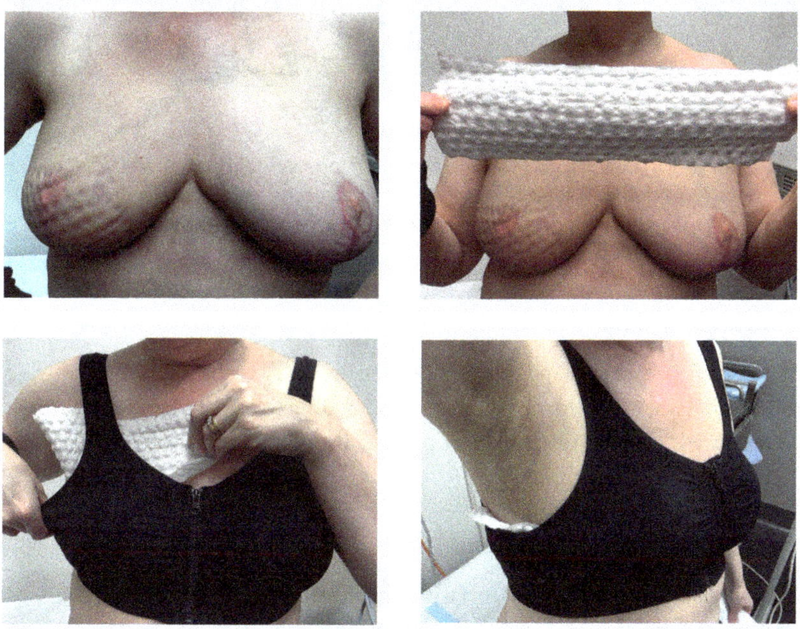

Figure 14.8

A compression vest with Mobiderm insert.

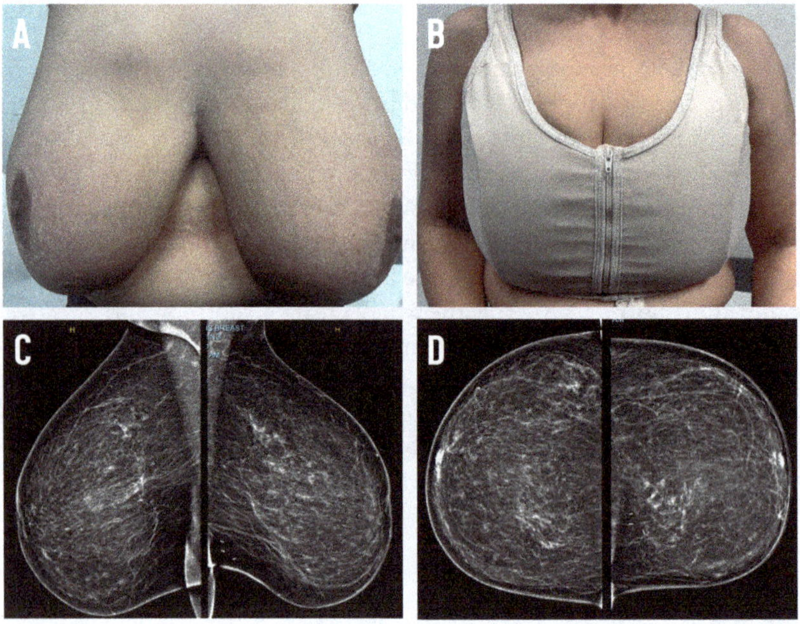

Figure 14.9

The patient from Figure 14.6 had significant improvement in breast swelling and heaviness (A), achieved with daily use of a compression bra (B). Mammogram images (C, D) highlight the reduction in skin thickness compared to her previous scans in Figure 14.5. The patient is using the Bellisse compression bra by Jobst.

Kinesiology tape

If you have breast oedema, kinesiology taping (KT) techniques may provide additional support, improve lymphatic drainage and reduce discomfort (**Figure 14.10**). You can find out more about KT in **Chapter 9**, Other Lymphoedema Therapies.

Pneumatic compression pumps

Sequential intermittent pneumatic compression (SIPC) pumps, discussed earlier in **Chapter 6**, Complex Lymphoedema Therapy, may also help manage oedema in the breast or chest wall. These devices use a vest-like garment to apply controlled pressure, promoting lymphatic flow to reduce swelling (see **Figure 6.8**). Sessions typically last up to an hour and can be done sitting or lying down. SIPC pumps may offer relief when used as part of a supervised tailored care plan.

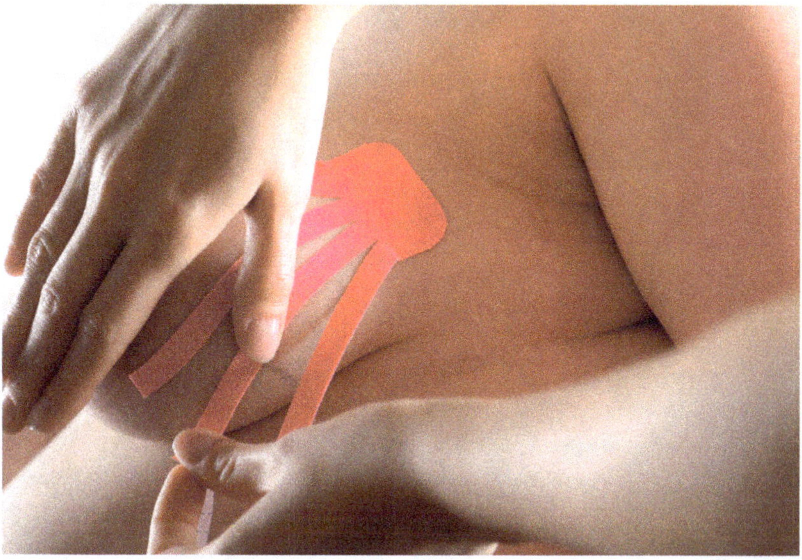

Figure 14.10

Kinesiology taping of the breast.

Lymphovenous anastomosis

In select cases, surgical intervention such as lymphovenous anastomosis (LVA) may be considered to treat breast oedema. LVA is a type of microsurgery involving the connection of lymphatic vessels to nearby blood vessels as a way to bypass a blockage and improve lymphatic drainage. I talk more about LVA in **Chapter 11**, Lymphatic Microsurgery.

CONCLUSION

Breast oedema is a complex condition that requires a multidisciplinary approach for effective management. Understanding its causes, utilising appropriate diagnostic techniques and implementing a comprehensive treatment plan tailored to your individual needs can do much to improve your quality of life if you are living with breast oedema. For therapists, an excellent article on breast oedema was written as collaboration between our ALERT team and Harvard University (Brunelle, 2024).

15

THE EMOTIONAL SIDE OF LYMPHOEDEMA

THE ROLLERCOASTER OF EMOTIONS

Discovering that you have lymphoedema can stir up a storm of emotions. You may feel angry, scared, sad or a mix of all three. After cancer treatment, it is common to feel a sense of relief and gratitude for overcoming cancer. However, to then be diagnosed with lymphoedema can be a real "kick in the guts", as one of my patients put it.

You may feel that sharing these emotions with your partner, family, or close friends is difficult at first. Alternatively, you may seek immediate support to help you untangle your feelings. Remember, it's natural for your emotions to ebb and flow, and sometimes catch you off guard. Many of the feelings you have may be similar to those you experienced at the time of your cancer diagnosis.

You may find the following tips helpful for seeking psychological support:

- Tell your treatment team how you're feeling – talk to your doctors, nurses or allied health professionals.
- In Australia, request a mental health care plan from your general practitioner to access subsidised sessions with a clinical psychologist.
- Engage with a lymphoedema support group.
- Reach out to understanding friends and family members.

Living with any chronic condition is challenging. It's crucial to give yourself time to come to terms with this new reality. A few of my patients are determined to simply get on with their lives; they accept the need to wear a compression garment when they go out, and have the strength of character to simply brush off any stares or intrusive questions they may encounter. For others, this new diagnosis can create intense anxiety and fear, leading them to explore many of the interventions covered in this book, including surgery.

For most people, living with a chronic condition will get easier with time. When I was diagnosed with Hodgkin's disease in 2017, I rode a rollercoaster of emotions and needed a lot of time off work. After multiple courses of chemotherapy, I ended up with the less visible side effect of peripheral neuropathy (pins and needles and numbness). I was annoyed at first, angry at my diagnosis, sad that I might not see my grandchildren grow up and frustrated that I had lost eight months of my life away from my patients and my research. However, with time, and with the help of my family, my friends and my faith, I was able to accept my situation and my new body. I have become more open about my experience and will sometimes share my story with a patient who is struggling with the tortures of their own diagnosis and treatment.

THE IMPACT OF LYMPHOEDEMA

In 2015, I worked closely with a great team in the Faculty of Business and Economics at Macquarie University, with support from Smith & Nephew, Breast Cancer Network Australia (BCNA) and the Australasian Lymphology Association (ALA), to produce a report on the psychosocial impact of lymphoedema.

In our report, we compared 209 patients with breast cancer alone to 152 patients with breast cancer and lymphoedema. As shown in **Table 15.1**, the patients who had lymphoedema in addition to breast cancer were worse off in every domain, from work to social life and their self-image. If you'd like to read more about our research, you can look at one of our published studies (Boyages, 2016, 2017; Kalfa, 2019).

IMPACT OF SIDE EFFECTS ON:	Breast cancer only	Breast cancer + lymphoedema
Work and career	51%	63%
Family life	59%	74%
Social life and leisure	38%	43%
Self-image	72%	79%

Table 15.1

Patients with breast cancer and lymphoedema experienced a higher impact on multiple life domains compared with having breast cancer alone (unpublished data).

In 2011, Professor Afaf Girgis surveyed 237 women with symptoms and signs of lymphoedema using the Lymphoedema Needs Questionnaire-Breast Cancer (LNQ-BC) tool, designed to assess the challenges faced by breast cancer patients who develop lymphoedema. The report found that patients with lymphoedema have several specific needs that require attention. The top three needs were:

- Ensuring doctors acknowledge lymphoedema as a serious condition
- Providing comprehensive education for medical professionals about lymphoedema and its associated challenges
- Ensuring doctors are willing to treat lymphoedema.

Other important needs included recognition and coverage by Medicare or private insurance, and information on alternative treatments. Up-to-date treatment options, early detection programs and well-informed healthcare professionals, including nurses, are essential. Patients also want information about available lymphoedema treatment centres and maintaining follow-up care (Girgis, 2011).

The latest BCNA State of the Nation report, published in June 2018, revealed that lymphoedema was the highest unmet information need, with 35% of participants highlighting a significant need for better resources on the condition (BCNA, 2018). This insight came from a comprehensive survey process with over 15,000 respondents, including 3,500 face-to-face consultations, a BCNA member survey with more than 10,000 respondents, a survey of another 2,000 participants on the financial impact of breast cancer, and input from health professionals specialising in breast cancer. These findings underscore the critical importance of addressing lymphoedema as a priority in breast cancer support and education.

SEEKING SUPPORT

Acknowledging your feelings is a significant step towards coping with your lymphoedema. Recognising that you're not alone in this journey is vital. It can be immensely beneficial to reach out for support through cancer support groups, counselling or connecting with fellow lymphoedema patients. You may find it helpful to look for an online support group at first. Sharing your experience and hearing other people's stories can provide comfort and understanding.

SELF-CARE AND MENTAL WELL-BEING

Caring for your mental health is as crucial as tending to your physical well-being. Find activities that bring you joy and help you to relax. You may wish to engage in mindfulness, meditation or gentle exercises to alleviate stress and anxiety. Surround yourself with friends and family who understand and support you.

INTIMACY AND RELATIONSHIPS

Lymphoedema can influence many aspects of your life, and one area where it can have a significant impact is your sexuality. Coping with physical changes and the emotional toll of lymphoedema can affect your self-esteem, body image and intimate relationships. It's essential to acknowledge these challenges and address them openly. In a study from the ALERT Centre, we recruited 17 women aged 38–67 who had mild to severe lymphoedema. We conducted and transcribed telephone interviews concerning sexual issues, and various themes emerged.

The women perceived that sexual concerns arising from lymphoedema exacerbated their concerns arising from breast cancer. Four interrelated factors determined the extent of lymphoedema's sexual impact: (a) swelling severity and location, (b) needing to wear a compression garment, (c) body image concerns raised by lymphoedema and breast cancer treatment, and (d) their sexual partner's acceptance and supportiveness. A supportive partner was instrumental in helping them overcome sexual issues caused by severe swelling and/or body image concerns. Few women reported being asked about sexual matters by any health professional, and most indicated that they were unwilling to discuss sexual concerns with health professionals, friends or family (Winch, 2015).

Communication with your partner is vital. Sharing your concerns, discussing physical changes and exploring ways to adapt to your new reality together can strengthen your relationship. You may find it valuable to seek professional counselling or sex therapy if you find these changes particularly challenging.

CHANGES IN BODY IMAGE AND SELF-ESTEEM

Lymphoedema may change the appearance and feel of your affected limb or breast. This can lead to a shift in how you perceive yourself, affecting your self-esteem.

Professor Kerry Sherman is a leading research psychologist from Macquarie University and I have worked with her for many years. With one of her

PhD students, Professor Sherman sought to understand how beliefs about lymphoedema, treatment effectiveness, and the ability to manage negative emotions influenced patients' feelings of depression, anxiety and stress. They also investigated whether age played a role in how body image disturbance affected psychological distress.

The study involved 166 Australian women with breast cancer-related lymphoedema recruited through a community-based breast cancer organisation and lymphoedema treatment clinics (Alcorso, 2016). The women completed an online survey which assessed their thoughts and beliefs about lymphoedema, the perceived effectiveness of their treatment, their ability to handle negative emotions and their level of body image disturbance. Additionally, the survey collected information on their levels of depression, anxiety and stress.

The results showed a clear link between negative beliefs about lymphoedema, perceived treatment effectiveness, the ability to manage negative emotions and the number of lymphoedema symptoms with higher levels of depression, anxiety and stress. Body image disturbance was particularly significant, as it was strongly associated with increased psychological distress. Interestingly, the study found that older women who experienced body image disturbance were more likely to suffer from depression and anxiety compared to their younger counterparts.

This study highlights the critical need for health professionals to recognise and address the psychological distress that can accompany a lymphoedema diagnosis. Women dealing with body image issues and those who believe their condition is uncontrollable are at a higher risk of mental health problems. It also suggests that older women may need additional support to cope with anxiety and depression related to body image disturbances. Overall, these insights underscore the importance of providing comprehensive care that addresses both the physical and emotional needs of women with lymphoedema.

It's important to remember that your body remains beautiful and unique, and self-acceptance is a journey. Seek support from the people you love, and from a therapist, psychologist or a support group. Although you may feel uncomfortable doing so, remember that you can raise any body image issues with your doctor, lymphoedema therapist or nurse.

Jela's Story

You hope to be one of the fortunate few not to develop the condition. You do all your occupational therapist tells you to do, and keep your fingers crossed. You put it out to the universe: please don't let me be in that 30% group. And then you read the percentage can be as high as 83%!

Well, I never did the "Why me?" when I got triple-negative breast cancer, and I was not going to question my bad luck as that slow, heavy swelling started in my right arm. So, living with lymphoedema is what I do. It's been ten years, and I deal with it daily.

Asked to share how it affects me, I can tell you that it's become my norm now. It's more of a challenge in summer when my arm swells and aches in the heat and humidity. I can't bring myself to wear sleeveless garments, so when shopping, I seek loose, blousy sleeves that disguise my bulging right arm. I know I must wear my compression sleeve, but sometimes I just say, "No way today! It's too hot!" – an ironic and not-so-smart decision, as the compression sleeve does help with the swelling.

Winter is a time of some relief. When that temperature starts dropping, the swelling and ache ease, and there are days, albeit few, when I forget I have this chronic condition. But summer is always around the corner. I was very self-conscious about my big arm, especially with the man in my life. But I've worked through it because this is me, and my daily regimen of self-massage, moisturising and using my fabulous massage machine is done openly in front of him. He even helps at times!

I am a breast cancer survivor, and I choose to see my big, bloated arm as a constant, beautiful reminder of my fortune. Maybe I should buy that lovely sleeveless dress I saw last week!

FINANCIAL CONSIDERATIONS

Lymphoedema may introduce financial challenges, which can add to the emotional stress you're under. Understanding the potential economic impacts and exploring strategies to manage them can help you navigate this aspect of your lymphoedema journey.

Lymphoedema often involves ongoing medical care, such as visits to specialists, the purchase of compression garments and the need to maintain necessary equipment. It's advisable to work with your healthcare team to understand the costs involved and explore health insurance or financial assistance options available to you. The ALA website includes a list of schemes and subsidies available in Australia for compression garments. Visit https://www.lymphoedema.org.au/about-lymphoedema/compression-garment-schemes/ or see **Useful websites**, page 174.

As part of our collaborative report in 2015, discussed earlier (see **Table 15.1**), we also examined the financial expense associated with having lymphoedema in addition to breast cancer. Both breast cancer and lymphoedema were found to cause significant out-of-pocket costs for patients. The results are summarised in **Table 15.2** below.

SURVEY ITEM	Breast cancer only	Breast cancer + lymphoedema
Breast cancer diagnosis affected me financially	67%	80%
Financial burden increased with lymphoedema diagnosis	–	56%

Table 15.2

Financial impact of breast cancer and lymphoedema on patients (Boyages, 2016).

As these results show, over half (56%) of the participants said that their lymphoedema diagnosis increased their financial burden, with costs rising as the severity of lymphoedema increased. Most of these costs (40.1%) were from buying compression garments (Boyages, 2016).

In the US, a recent study on the cost-effectiveness of liposuction for advanced lymphoedema was conducted at two leading lymphoedema centres (Bloom, 2022). The research compared patients who underwent debulking surgery with those using conservative management. By analysing procedural costs, **quality-adjusted life years (QALYs)** and overall healthcare expenses, the study assessed which approach provided better value.

The results showed that, while liposuction surgery had an initial cost of about $8,753 (in US dollars), it significantly reduced long-term healthcare expenses by improving patient outcomes and preventing the need for ongoing care. By contrast, conservative management incurred higher lifetime costs of approximately $83,240. The analysis demonstrated that surgery provided better QALYs for the patient and was more cost-effective overall (Bloom, 2022).

Financial concerns can contribute to emotional stress. Remember that it's normal to feel anxious about financial matters, but seeking support from a financial counsellor or social worker can provide guidance and alleviate some of your worries.

WORK AND CAREER

Lymphoedema may affect your ability to work in certain professions, or it may require workplace accommodations in some cases. Discuss your situation with your employer and consider seeking advice from vocational rehabilitation services if necessary. It is essential that you understand your rights and legal protections in the workplace regarding your lymphoedema.

WHAT ELSE COULD HELP?

In addition to standard treatments, integrative therapies like acupuncture and yoga, which can aid with tissue flexibility and stress management, have gained popularity. There is some supporting evidence to show that they may be beneficial for people with lymphoedema or those at risk.

In 1995, when I was the founding director of the Westmead Breast Cancer Institute, I implemented many support programs for our patients. One of my staff members suggested we start a yoga program for our patients with breast cancer. I was a little hesitant at first, but it became one of our most attended programs – after starting with a daytime class, we had to add an after-hours class due to the popularity. The benefit of exercise, stretching, balance, mindfulness and flexibility cannot be overstated. Furthermore, connecting with fellow breast cancer and lymphoedema survivors, reassuring you that you are not alone, can be extremely therapeutic.

A meta-analysis by Freguia (2024) from Bologna University summarised the benefits of yoga for breast cancer survivors with lymphoedema. This review looked at three key randomised controlled trials, encompassing a total of 96 patients. The findings highlighted that yoga, when integrated into routine care, improved the participants' quality of life by reducing fatigue, pain and insomnia and enhancing physical function. Specifically, yoga contributed to better shoulder strength and spinal mobility, and reduced tissue stiffness. However, it did not consistently reduce limb swelling.

The reviewed studies identified that yoga, especially when tailored to individual needs and involving both in-person and home sessions, can play a beneficial role in comprehensive lymphoedema management. These findings underline the potential of combining conventional treatment with integrative practices to support both the physical and emotional aspects of recovery.

CONCLUSION

When I began working in breast oncology 40 years ago, lymphoedema was recognised as an unfortunate consequence of cancer treatment. We recorded its presence but had little treatment or advice to offer. Today, fewer people face a lymphoedema diagnosis, thanks to less invasive surgical and radiation techniques and a deeper understanding of minimising harm to the lymph nodes. Screening and early intervention for subclinical lymphoedema have also reduced its incidence and severity.

As you gain knowledge and work with dedicated lymphoedema therapists, you'll discover tools and techniques that enable you to lead a full, active life. The stories in this book demonstrate that with commitment, self-compassion and the right support, lymphoedema doesn't have to stand in the way of achieving your dreams or embracing life's opportunities.

My father lost his hand at the age of 24 while clearing a rubbish dump for the British military administration in Rhodes, Greece. His handwritten diary reveals his despair as he travelled to Australia with "no wife, no hand, no job, and no hope". I remember him hiding his stump and telling me about his workmates teasing him in that cheeky Australian way (he eventually didn't mind being called "Leftie").

He felt the shame and stigma of being different, perhaps even feeling inferior. I recognise the intensity of some of these feelings and remember dad when patients tell me, “I can hide my mastectomy scar, but not my arm in a compression sleeve.”

Over time, he grew more resilient, eventually obtaining his driving licence, driving a car with his left arm with four gears on the floor, and painting the outside of our house while holding a paint can on his left arm and balancing on a ladder. He played with us as kids, tickling us with his stump in a game we called “Give us the stump, Dad!” Though he was smart – dux of his class each year of his seven years at school – the war intervened, leaving him orphaned at 13 and without further education.

He became a cleaner, a proud Australian, and a Qantas employee. In his diary, he wrote, “I wish someone had encouraged me while I was coming to Australia, full of apprehension, and said to me: ‘Do not worry, mate. In 35 years, you’ll have three professional children and seven highly educated, adoring grandchildren’.” We never know what the future holds.

Looking forward, advancements in research, treatment and awareness are creating a brighter future for people living with lymphoedema. We are entering a new era where innovative surgical techniques, better diagnostic tools, and integrative therapies are becoming more accessible. I am confident that there are more innovations on the horizon – ones that will not only reduce harm to the lymphatic system but also offer more sophisticated, targeted therapies. Perhaps, with continued research, lymphoedema may even be cured one day.

Remember, lymphoedema doesn’t define you – like my father, you may have your ups and downs, but with time your strength, resilience, adaptability and optimism will become stronger. Take small steps at first, remembering to care for your mind and body. Build relationships with family, old friends and new friends, and remember that the best things in life are free. God bless.

Endnotes

CREDITS

Editor: Felicity Sutton

Design and production: John and Yolande Bull, Publishing Art Australia

Additional editing: Philippa Sutton

Images and graphics:

Cover: John Bull, Publishing Art Australia

Author photo, previous book covers, BC Publishing logo: Copyright BC Publishing

Figures **1.1** [Alila Medical Media], **4.1** [stockyimages], **4.9** [Tyler Olson], **6.1**, [Petia_is], **7.1** [Prostock-studio], **7.2A** [Zay Nyi-Nyi], **7.2B** [sruilk], **12.1** [Ronald Rampsch], **12.2** [michaeljung], **12.3** [Bocharev Photography], **13.1** [249 Anurak], **14.10** [Doro Guzenda]: Used under licence from Shutterstock

Figures **1.2**, **1.3**, **2.1**, **4.7**, **4.8**: Copyright Hiroo Suami

Figure **2.3**: Copyright Håkan Brorson

Figures **2.2**, **3.1**, **3.2**, **4.2**, **4.3**, **4.6**, **5.1**, **8.5**, **9.2**, **13.2**, **14.1–14.5**, **14.8**, **14.9**: Copyright BC Publishing, with patient permission

Figures **4.4**, **5.2**: Copyright ImpediMed Limited, with permission

Figures **4.5**, **4.10**, **6.2–6.4**, **10.1**, **10.2**,**10.4**, **14.6**, **14.7**: With permission from ALERT Centre (including patient permission)

Figures **6.5**, **8.1**, **8.2**: Copyright Medi Australia, with permission

Figure **6.6**, **10.3**: Copyright Haddenham Healthcare Limited [2025]. HADDENHAM® / COMFIWAVE® is a registered trademark of Haddenham Healthcare Limited and used with permission. All rights reserved.

Figure **6.7**, **6.8**: Copyright Medi Rent Australia

Figure **8.3**: Copyright Essity-Jobst

Figure **8.4**, **12.4**: Copyright LympheDIVAS

Figure **9.1**: Copyright Lymphatic Solutions, with permission (https://lymphaticsolutions.com.au/)

ABBREVIATIONS

ALA: Australasian Lymphology Association

ALERT: Australian Lymphoedema Education Research and Treatment

A/Prof: Associate Professor

BCI: [Westmead] Breast Cancer Institute

BCNA: Breast Cancer Network of Australia

BLS: British Lymphology Society

CLT: Complex lymphoedema therapy

COSA: Clinical Oncology Society of Australia

CT: Computed tomography

FBC: Full blood count

ICG: Indocyanine green

LANA: Lymphology Association of North America

LE&RN: Lymphatic Education and Research Network

LNT: Lymph node transfer

LVA: Lymphovenous anastomosis

MLD: Manual lymphatic drainage

MLS: Multi-wave locked system

MRI: Magnetic resonance imaging

SIPC: Sequential intermittent pneumatic compression

GLOSSARY

Adipose tissue: Fat cells storing energy in the body.

Anastomosis: Surgical connection made between two structures in the body (such as blood vessels).

Antibacterial: Designed to kill or prevent the growth of bacteria, e.g. treating a bacterial infection on the skin.

Antifungal: Designed to kill or prevent the growth of fungal organisms, e.g. treating a fungal infection on the skin.

Axilla: The armpit area.

Axillary lymph node dissection (ALND): Surgical procedure to remove lymph nodes from under the arm. Also known as axillary dissection, axillary clearance, or axillary lymphadenectomy.

Bioimpedance spectroscopy (BIS): A non-invasive clinical test that measures body composition, such as water and fat content, by passing a safe electric current through the body tissue.

Breast oedema: Swelling of the breast tissue.

Cellulitis: Bacterial skin infection causing redness, swelling, and pain.

Chronic lymphoedema: Moderate or severe persistent lymphoedema; long-term swelling in the body's tissues from a build-up of fluid.

Complete decongestive therapy (CDT): Treatment approach for lymphoedema involving manual lymphatic drainage and compression therapy. Known as complex lymphoedema therapy in some countries.

Complex lymphoedema therapy (CLT): Comprehensive treatment method for lymphoedema including skin care, compression techniques, exercise and manual lymphatic drainage.

Deep fascia: Dense connective tissue covering muscles and organs.

Dermal backflow: A condition where lymphatic fluid leaks into the skin due to impaired lymphatic drainage, leading to swelling and skin changes.

Diuretic: Medication promoting increased urine production and fluid elimination.

Doff: To remove a piece of clothing.

Don: To put on a piece of clothing.

Endothelial cells: Layer of cells lining the lymphatic vessels that regulate the transport of lymph, immune cells and waste products throughout the lymphatic system. They also maintain tissue fluid balance, immune response and the formation of new lymphatic vessels.

Erysipelas: Acute bacterial infection causing red, swollen, and painful skin.

Fibrosis: Scarring caused by formation of excess fibrous connective tissue.

Indocyanine green lymphography (ICG): Imaging technique using fluorescent indocyanine green dye to visualise lymphatic vessels.

Inflammatory breast cancer: Aggressive form of breast cancer with symptoms including redness, swelling, and warmth.

Interval lymph node: Lymph node that lymphatic fluid passes through on its way from a primary site of lymphatic drainage (such as a limb) to a more centrally located node (regional lymph node) to be drained.

Intravenous (IV): Within or administered into a vein, such as administration of medication or fluids directly into a vein.

Kinesiology tape (KT): Elastic therapeutic tape used for support and rehabilitation.

Liposuction: Surgical procedure to remove excess fat from the body.

Low-level laser therapy (LLLT): Treatment using low-intensity lasers for tissue healing and pain relief.

Lymph: A colourless fluid containing white blood cells, which bathes the tissues and drains through the lymphatic system into the bloodstream.

Lymph node: Small, bean-shaped structure responsible for filtering lymph and fighting infections.

Lymph node transfer (LNT): Surgical procedure involving the transfer of lymph nodes to improve lymphatic drainage.

Lymphatic capillaries: The smallest lymphatic vessels, found in tissues all over the body. The capillaries exist in the spaces between cells and are responsible for draining and processing extracellular fluid. Also called lymph capillaries or initial lymphatics.

Lymphatic system: Network of vessels, nodes, and organs responsible for fluid drainage and immune response.

Lymphangitis: Inflammation of lymphatic vessels.

Lymphoedema rubra: Blanching redness of lymphoedema-affected skin caused by inflammation of blood vessels, that is often mistaken for cellulitis.

Lymphoedema therapist: A healthcare professional specially trained in the diagnosis, treatment and management of lymphoedema. They can come from various clinical backgrounds, including physiotherapy, occupational therapy or nursing.

Lymphorrhoea: Leaking of lymph through the surface of the skin.

Lymphovenous anastomosis (LVA): Surgical connection between lymphatic and venous systems.

Macrophages: Specialised white blood cells that help remove dead cells, fight infection, and reduce inflammation in your body.

Magnetic resonance imaging (MRI): Diagnostic imaging technique using magnetic fields and radio waves.

Manual lymphatic drainage (MLD): A specialised massage technique designed to stimulate lymph flow, redirecting fluid to healthy lymph nodes or alternative drainage pathways when blockages occur.

Mitochondria: Small structures within cells that produce energy, essential for various cellular functions and overall health.

Moisture meter: Device measuring moisture levels in the skin.

Near-infrared fluorescent lymphography: Imaging technique using near-infrared light to visualise lymphatic vessels (see also ICG lymphography).

Oedema: Abnormal accumulation of fluid in body tissues causing swelling.

Peau d'orange: Skin condition characterised by a dimpled appearance resembling orange peel, associated with blocked lymphatic vessels.

Perometer: Device measuring limb volume derived from multiple circumference measurements.

PET-CT scan: Diagnostic imaging technique combining the methods of positron-emission tomography (PET) and computed tomography (CT) in the same scan.

Placebo: Inactive substance given as a control in clinical trials.

Platelet count: The average level of platelets in your blood as shown on a blood test. Platelets are tiny blood cells responsible for helping the blood to clot.

Pitting: Indentation left on the skin after pressure is applied for at least a minute.

Primary lymphoedema: Inherited condition causing lymphatic system abnormalities and swelling.

Quality-adjusted life years (QALYs): A measure that combines the length of time and quality of life that a treatment provides. One QALY equals one year of life in perfect health. Higher QALYs indicate better health outcomes and more effective treatments.

Radiation: Treatment using high-energy rays to destroy cancer cells.

Ready-to-wear garment: Pre-made compression garment available to purchase in standard sizes, as opposed to being custom-made for an individual. Also called over-the-counter garment.

Regional lymph node: Lymph node that drains lymph from a specific body region, often the first site where cancer spreads. For example, cancers of the hand, arm or breast may spread to regional lymph nodes in the axilla.

Secondary lymphoedema: Lymphoedema caused by an underlying condition or treatment.

Sequential intermittent pneumatic compression (SIPC): Therapy using inflatable garments to promote lymphatic flow.

Sentinel lymph node: The first lymph node to receive drainage from a particular body region, such as the breast or arm. As the first place where cancer cells are likely to spread, it is often examined and/or treated.

Seroma: A collection of fluid that can build up under the skin after surgery.

Stratum corneum: The outermost skin layer, made of dead cells, forming a protective barrier against and preserving moisture.

Supraclavicular fossa: Depression above the collarbone where blood vessels, nerves and lymph nodes are located.

Systematic review: A detailed and organised summary of all the research on a particular topic, where scientists gather and analyse data from multiple studies to draw more reliable conclusions.

Thoracic duct: Major lymphatic vessel in the chest that drains lymph into the bloodstream.

Venules: Small blood vessels connecting capillaries to veins.

USEFUL WEBSITES

Websites referenced in text (in order of appearance)

RESOURCE	Link	Page
BCI patient information on post-surgery shoulder care:	https://www.bci.org.au/breast-cancer-information/fact-sheets/shoulder-care/	53
COSA position statement on exercise:	https://www.cosa.org.au/advocacy/position-statements/exercise-in-cancer-care/	65
ALA supplier list:	https://www.lymphoedema.org.au/education-&-resources/lymphoedema-supplier-list/	82
LE&RN Centers of Excellence:	https://lymphaticnetwork.org/centers-of-excellence	104
BLS guidelines on vaccination:	https://www.thebls.com/public/uploads/documents/document-15921697117874.pdf	122
Summary of 2024 LANA recommendations:	https://link.springer.com/article/10.1007/s12032-024-02510-6/figures/1	128
BLS guidelines on cellulitis:	https://www.thebls.com/public/uploads/documents/document-66331665737684.pdf	122
ALA consensus guideline on cellulitis:	https://www.lymphoedema.org.au/about-lymphoedema/consensus-guideline/	82
Compression garment schemes/subsidies (Australia/New Zealand):	https://www.lymphoedema.org.au/about-lymphoedema/compression-garment-schemes/	82

Professional bodies, general information and support

RESOURCE	Link
American Cancer Society – Lymphedema:	https://www.cancer.org/cancer/managing-cancer/side-effects/swelling/lymphedema.html
Australasian Lymphology Association (ALA):	https://www.lymphoedema.org.au
ALA National Lymphoedema Practitioners Register:	https://www.lymphoedema.org.au/accreditation-nlpr/find-a-practitioner/
Better Health Channel – Lymphoedema:	https://www.betterhealth.vic.gov.au/health/conditionsandtreatments/lymphoedema
Breast Cancer Network Australia (BCNA) – Lymphoedema:	https://www.bcna.org.au/resource-hub/articles/lymphoedema/
BreastCancer.org – Lymphedema:	https://www.breastcancer.org/treatment-side-effects/lymphedema
British Lymphology Society (BLS):	https://www.thebls.com/
Cancer Council Australia – Lymphoedema:	https://www.cancer.org.au/cancer-information/after-a-diagnosis/after-cancer-treatment/lymphoedema
Health Direct – Lymphoedema:	https://www.healthdirect.gov.au/lymphoedema
Lymphatic Education and Research Network (LE&RN):	https://lymphaticnetwork.org
Lymphcare Australia:	https://www.lymphcare.com.au
Lymphoedema Association of Australia (LAA):	https://www.lymphaustralia.org.au
Lymphoedema Support Network (LSN):	https://www.lymphoedema.org

Professional bodies, general information and support cont'd

RESOURCE	Link
Lymphology Association of North America (LANA):	https://www.clt-lana.org
LANA – Find a practitioner:	https://www.clt-lana.org/therapists
Macmillan Cancer Support – Lymphoedema:	https://www.macmillan.org.uk/cancer-information-and-support/impacts-of-cancer/lymphoedema
Macquarie University – ALERT:	https://www.mqhealth.org.au/services/find-a-service/lymphoedema-clinic
Mayo Clinic – Lymphedema:	https://www.mayoclinic.org/diseases-conditions/lymphedema/symptoms-causes/syc-20374682
Memorial Sloan Kettering Cancer Center – Lymphedema and Breast Cancer:	https://www.mskcc.org/cancer-care/patient-education/facts-about-lymphedema-and-breast
National Cancer Institute – Lymphedema:	https://www.cancer.gov/about-cancer/treatment/side-effects/lymphedema
National Lymphedema Network (NLN):	https://lymphnet.org/
The Lymphie Life:	https://thelymphielife.com/
Westmead Breast Cancer Institute (BCI):	https://www.bci.org.au/

REFERENCES

Akita, Shinsuke, et al. Early detection of lymphatic disorder and treatment for lymphedema following breast cancer. Plastic and Reconstructive Surgery 138.2 (2016): 192e-202e.

Alcorso, Jessica, and Kerry A. Sherman. Factors associated with psychological distress in women with breast cancer-related lymphoedema. Psycho-Oncology 25.7 (2016): 865-872.

Ali, Saba M., and Gil Yosipovitch. Skin pH: from basic science to basic skin care. Acta Dermato-Venereologica 93.3 (2013): 261-267.

Armer, Jane M. The problem of post-breast cancer lymphedema: impact and measurement issues. Cancer Investigation 23.1 (2005): 76-83.

Baxter, G. David, et al. Low level laser therapy (photobiomodulation therapy) for breast cancer-related lymphedema: a systematic review. BMC Cancer 17.1 (2017): 1-13.

Bloom, Joshua A., et al. Power-assisted liposuction for lymphedema: a cost-utility analysis. Plastic and Reconstructive Surgery – Global Open 10.11 (2022): e4671.

Boughey, Judy C., et al. Risk factors associated with breast lymphedema. Annals of Surgical Oncology 21 (2014): 1202-1208.

Boyages, John, et al. Early breast cancer: cosmetic and functional results after treatment by conservative techniques. Australian and New Zealand Journal of Surgery 58.2 (1988): 111-121.

Boyages, John, et al. Worse and worse off: the impact of lymphedema on work and career after breast cancer. Springerplus 5.1 (2016): 657.

Boyages, John, et al. Financial cost of lymphedema borne by women with breast cancer. Psycho-Oncology 26.6 (2017): 849-855.

Boyages, John, et al. The ALERT model of care for the assessment and personalized management of patients with lymphoedema. British Journal of Surgery 107.3 (2020): 238-247.

Boyages, John, et al. Weight gain and lymphedema after breast cancer treatment: avoiding the catch-22? Lymphatic Research and Biology 20.4 (2022): 409-416.

Boyages, John, et al. Axillary treatment and chronic breast cancer-related lymphedema: implications for prospective surveillance and intervention from a randomized controlled trial. JCO Oncology Practice (2023): OP-23.

Breast Cancer Network Australia [**BCNA**]. State of the nation. Breast Cancer Network Australia (2018): https://bcna-dxp.azureedge.net/media/uoqnz1kw/bcna_state-of-the-nation-report_2018.pdf

British Lymphology Society [**BLS**]. Guidelines on the management of cellulitis in lymphoedema. British Lymphology Society and the Lymphoedema Support Network (2022): https://www.thebls.com/documents-library/guidelines-on-the-management-of-cellulitis-in-lymphoedema

BLS. Guidelines on Covid-19 and flu vaccinations for people with lymphoedema. British Lymphology Society and the Lymphoedema Support Network (2023): https://www.thebls.com/documents-library/guidance-on-covid-19-and-flu-vaccinations-for-people-with-lymphoedema

Brorson, Håkan, et al. Breast cancer-related chronic arm lymphedema is associated with excess adipose and muscle tissue. Lymphatic Research and Biology 7.1 (2009): 3-10.

Brorson, Håkan. From lymph to fat: liposuction as a treatment for complete reduction of lymphedema. International Journal of Lower Extremity Wounds 11.1 (2012): 10-19.

Brorson, Håkan. Complete reduction of arm lymphedema following breast cancer – a prospective twenty-one years' study. Plastic and Reconstructive Surgery 136.4S (2015): 134-135.

Brorson, Håkan, et al. Complete reduction of leg lymphedema in 126 patients with liposuction without recurrence – 20 years' follow-up. Plastic and Reconstructive Surgery – Global Open 10.10S (2022): 130-131.

Brunelle, Cheryl L., et al. Patients who report cording after breast cancer surgery are at higher risk of lymphedema: results from a large prospective screening cohort. Journal of Surgical Oncology 122.2 (2020): 155-163.

Brunelle, Cheryl L., and Alphonse G. Taghian. The important role of nighttime compression in breast cancer–related lymphedema treatment. Cancer 128.3 (2022): 458-460.

Brunelle, Cheryl L., et al. Breast lymphedema following breast-conserving treatment for breast cancer: current status and future directions. Breast Cancer Research and Treatment 204.2 (2024a): 193-222.

Brunelle, Cheryl L., et al. Evidence-based recommendations regarding risk reduction practices for people at risk of or with breast cancer-related lymphedema: consensus from an expert panel. Medical Oncology 41.11 (2024b): 1-5.

Cavezzi, Attilio, et al. Lymphedema and nutrition: a review. Veins and Lymphatics 8.1 (2019): 8220.

Chien, Tsai-Ju, et al. The effect of acupuncture in breast cancer–related lymphoedema (BCRL): a systematic review and meta-analysis. Integrative Cancer Therapies 18 (2019): 1-9.

Cho, Kye Hee, et al. Feasibility of bioimpedance analysis to assess the outcome of complex decongestive therapy in cancer treatment-related lymphedema. Frontiers in Oncology 10 (2020): 111.

Chua, Boon, et al. Is there a role for axillary dissection for patients with operable breast cancer in this era of conservatism? ANZ Journal of Surgery 72.11 (2002): 786-792.

Clarke, Daniel, et al. Breast edema following staging axillary node dissection in patients with breast carcinoma treated by radical radiotherapy. Cancer 49.11 (1982): 2295-2299.

Cormie, Prue, et al. Clinical Oncology Society of Australia position statement on exercise in cancer care. Medical Journal of Australia 209.4 (2018): 184-187.

Czerniec, Sharon A., et al. Assessment of breast cancer-related lymphedema: a comparison of moisture meter and spot bioimpedance measurement. Lymphatic Research and Biology 13.1 (2015): 10-19.

Deen, Afka, et al. Chemical composition and health benefits of coconut oil: an overview. Journal of the Science of Food and Agriculture 101.6 (2021): 2182-2193.

Devoogdt, Nele, et al. The effectiveness of fluoroscopy-guided manual lymph drainage as part of decongestive lymphatic therapy on the superficial lymphatic architecture in patients with breast cancer-related lymphoedema: a randomised controlled trial. Cancers 15.5 (2023): 1545.

De Vrieze, Tessa, et al. Does manual lymphatic drainage add value in reducing suprafascial fluid accumulation and skin elasticity in patients with breast cancer–related lymphedema? Physical Therapy 102.12 (2022): pzac137.

Dionyssiou, Dimitrios, et al. A randomized control study of treating secondary stage II breast cancer-related lymphoedema with free lymph node transfer. Breast Cancer Research and Treatment 156 (2016): 73-79.

Ferguson, Chantal M., et al. Impact of ipsilateral blood draws, injections, blood pressure measurements, and air travel on the risk of lymphedema for patients treated for breast cancer. Journal of Clinical Oncology 34.7 (2016): 691.

Ferrandez, Jean-Claude, and Daniel Serin. Rééducation et cancer du sein, 1st edn. Masson, 1996.

Fife, Caroline E., et al. Skin and wound care in lymphedema patients: a taxonomy, primer, and literature review. Advances in skin & wound care 30.7 (2017): 305-318.

Freguia, Sara, et al. Closing the gaps: an integrative review of yoga's benefits for lymphedema in breast cancer survivors. Life 14.8 (2024): 999.

Fritz, Stephanie A., et al. Effectiveness of measures to eradicate Staphylococcus aureus carriage in patients with community-associated skin and soft-tissue infections: a randomized trial. Infection Control & Hospital Epidemiology 32.9 (2011): 872-880.

Gáspár, Lajos. Professor Endre Mester, the father of photobiomodulation. Journal of Laser Dentistry 17.3 (2009): 146-148.

Girgis, Afaf, et al. Priorities for women with lymphoedema after treatment for breast cancer: population based cohort study. British Medical Journal (2011): 342.

Granoff, Melisa D., et al. A 4-year institutional experience of immediate lymphatic reconstruction. Plastic and Reconstructive Surgery 152.5 (2023): 773e-778e.

Greene, Arin K. Myths associated with lymphedema. Lymphedema. Springer, Cham, 2015, 45-50.

Haesler, E. Evidence summary: single modality treatment of lymphoedema: manual lymphatic drainage. Wound Practice & Research: Journal of the Australian Wound Management Association 24.2 (2016a): 116-118.

Haesler, E. Evidence summary: managing lymphoedema: complex lymphoedema therapy.Wound Practice & Research: Journal of the Australian Wound Management Association 24.2 (2016b): 121-124.

Heller, Danielle R., et al. Quality of life after axillary lymph node dissection among racial and ethnic minority women. JAMA Surgery 159.6 (2024): 668-676.

Hoffner, Mattias, et al. Lymphedema leads to fat deposition in muscle and decreased muscle/water volume after liposuction: a magnetic resonance imaging study. Lymphatic Research and Biology 16.2 (2018a): 174-181.

Hoffner, Mattias, et al. Liposuction gives complete reduction of arm lymphedema following breast cancer treatment – a 5-year prospective study in 105 patients without recurrence. Plastic and Reconstructive Surgery – Global Open 6.8 (2018b): e1912.

Iannello, Christina, and Marcy K. Biller. Management of edema using simple manual lymphatic drainage techniques for hand and upper extremity patients. Journal of Hand Therapy 33.4 (2020): 616-619.

International Society of Lymphology [ISL]. The diagnosis and treatment of peripheral lymphedema: 2023 consensus document of the International Society of Lymphology. Lymphology 56.4 (2023): 133-151.

Jakes, Adam D., and Chris Twelves. Breast cancer-related lymphoedema and venepuncture: a review and evidence-based recommendations. Breast Cancer Research and Treatment 154 (2015): 455-461.

Johansson, Karin, et al. Axillary web syndrome: evidence for lymphatic origin with thrombosis. Lymphatic Research and Biology 18.4 (2020): 329-332.

Johnson, Anna Rose, et al. Lymphedema incidence after axillary lymph node dissection: quantifying the impact of radiation and the lymphatic microsurgical preventive healing approach. Annals of Plastic Surgery 82.4S (2019): S234-S241.

Johnson, Anna Rose, et al. Evaluating the impact of immediate lymphatic reconstruction for the surgical prevention of lymphedema. Plastic and Reconstructive Surgery 147.3 (2021): 373e-381e.

Kalfa, Senia, et al. Work experiences of Australian cancer survivors with lymphoedema: a qualitative study. Health & Social Care in the Community 27.4 (2019): 848-855.

Karlsson, Tobias, et al. Liposuction and controlled compression therapy reduce the erysipelas incidence in primary and secondary lymphedema. Plastic and Reconstructive Surgery – Global Open 10.5 (2022): e4314.

Karlsson, Tobias, et al. Liposuction for advanced lymphedema in a multidisciplinary team setting in Australia: 5-year follow-up. Plastic and Reconstructive Surgery 153.2 (2024): 482-491.

Karu, Tiina. Ten lectures on basic science of laser phototherapy. Prima Books, 2007.

Kilbreath, Sharon L., et al. Effect of air travel on lymphedema risk in women with history of breast cancer. Breast cancer research and treatment 120 (2010): 649-654.

Kilbreath, Sharon L., et al. Reduction of breast lymphoedema secondary to breast cancer: a randomised controlled exercise trial. Breast Cancer Research and Treatment 184 (2020): 459-467.

Koelmeyer, Louise A., et al. Early surveillance is associated with less incidence and severity of breast cancer–related lymphedema compared with a traditional referral model of care. Cancer 125.6 (2019): 854-862.

Koelmeyer, Louise A., et al. Personalizing conservative lymphedema management using indocyanine green-guided manual lymphatic drainage. Lymphatic Research and Biology 19.1 (2021): 56-65.

Koelmeyer, Louise A., et al. Risk factors for breast cancer–related lymphedema in patients undergoing 3 years of prospective surveillance with intervention. Cancer 128.18 (2022): 3408-3415.

Koshima, Isao, et al. Paraumbilical perforator flap without deep inferior epigastric vessels. Plastic and Reconstructive Surgery 102.4 (1998): 1052-1057.

Kwan, Marilyn L., et al. Exercise in patients with lymphedema: a systematic review of the contemporary literature. Journal of Cancer Survivorship 5.4 (2011): 320-336.

Lee, D., et al. Liposuction of postmastectomy arm lymphedema decreases the incidence of erysipelas. Lymphology 49.2 (2016): 85-92.

Leidenius, Marjut, et al. Motion restriction and axillary web syndrome after sentinel node biopsy and axillary clearance in breast cancer. The American Journal of Surgery 185.2 (2003): 127-130.

Levy, Adam S., et al. Lymphatic microsurgical preventive healing approach for the primary prevention of lymphedema: a 4-year follow-up. Plastic and Reconstructive Surgery 151.2 (2023): 413-420.

Liu, N. F., and W. Olszewski. The influence of local hyperthermia on lymphedema and lymphedematous skin of the human leg. Lymphology 26.1 (1993): 28-37.

Mahmood, Dania, et al. Clinical application of low-level laser therapy (photo-biomodulation therapy) in the management of breast cancer-related lymphedema: a systematic review. BMC Cancer 22.1 (2022): 937.

McGinity, Erin N., et al. The current state of lymphedema surgery. Lymphatics 2.4 (2024): 212-227.

McNeely, Margaret L., et al. Nighttime compression supports improved self-management of breast cancer–related lymphedema: a multicenter randomized controlled trial. Cancer 128.3 (2022): 587-596.

Meuli, Joachim N., et al. Outcomes after microsurgical treatment of lymphedema: a systematic review and meta-analysis. International Journal of Surgery 109.5 (2023): 1360-1372.

Moffatt, C. J., et al. A preliminary randomized controlled study to determine the application frequency of a new lymphoedema bandaging system. British Journal of Dermatology 166.3 (2012): 624-632.

Mondor, Henri. Tronculite sous-cutanée subaiguë de la paroi thoracique antérolatérale. Mémoires de l'Académie de Chirurgie 65 (1939): 1271-1278.

Moskovitz, Alexander H., et al. Axillary web syndrome after axillary dissection. The American Journal of Surgery 181.5 (2001): 434-439.

Naoum, George E., et al. Quantifying the impact of axillary surgery and nodal irradiation on breast cancer–related lymphedema and local tumor control: long-term results from a prospective screening trial. Journal of Clinical Oncology 38.29 (2020): 3430.

Newton, Robert U., et al. Clinical Oncology Society of Australia position statement on exercise in cancer care. The Medical Journal of Australia 210.1 (2019): 54.

Ngo, Quan D., et al. Vascularized lymph node transfer for patients with breast cancer-related lymphedema can potentially reduce the burden of ongoing conservative management. Lymphatic Research and Biology 18.4 (2020): 357-364.

O'Brien, Bernard M., et al. Microlymphaticovenous anastomoses for obstructive lymphedema. Plastic and Reconstructive Surgery 60.2 (1977): 197-211.

Otero, Violeta, et al. Kinesio taping versus compression garments for treating breast cancer–related lymphedema: a randomized, cross-over, controlled trial. Clinical Rehabilitation 33.12 (2019): 1887-1897.

Pigott, Amanda, et al. It was just mind blowing to be honest: a qualitative phenomenological study exploring cancer survivor's experiences of indocyanine green lymphography used to inform lymphedema therapy management. Supportive Care in Cancer 29.11 (2021): 6389-6397.

Quirke, M., et al. Risk factors for non-purulent leg cellulitis: a systematic review and meta-analysis. British Journal of Dermatology 177.2 (2017): 382-394.

Raff, Adam B., and Daniela Kroshinsky. Cellulitis: a review. JAMA 316.3 (2016): 325-337.

Ridner, Sheila H. Quality of life and a symptom cluster associated with breast cancer treatment-related lymphedema, Supportive Care in Cancer 13: (2005): 904-911.

Ridner, Sheila H., et al. A randomized trial evaluating bioimpedance spectroscopy versus tape measurement for the prevention of lymphedema following treatment for breast cancer: interim analysis. Annals of Surgical Oncology 26.10 (2019): 3250-3259.

Ridner, Sheila H., et al. Advanced pneumatic compression for treatment of lymphedema of the head and neck: a randomized wait-list controlled trial. Supportive Care in Cancer 29 (2021): 795-803.

Ridner, Sheila H., et al. A comparison of bioimpedance spectroscopy or tape measure triggered compression intervention in chronic breast cancer lymphedema prevention. Lymphatic Research and Biology 20.6 (2022): 618-628.

Rockson, Stanley G., et al. Pilot studies demonstrate the potential benefits of antiinflammatory therapy in human lymphedema. JCI Insight 3.20 (2018): e123775.

Rönkä, Riitta H., et al. Breast lymphedema after breast conserving treatment. Acta Oncologica 43.6 (2004): 551-557.

Ryan, Terence J. The skin as a barrier: what does it mean when it fails when lymphoedema is present? Journal of Lymphodema 8.1 (2013).

Ryan, Terence J. Care of oedematous skin in a resource-poor environment: a commentary of practice strategies to address a global community need. Wound Practice & Research: Journal of the Australian Wound Management Association 25.3 (2017): 134-137.

Sanal-Toprak, C., et al. The efficacy of intermittent pneumatic compression as a substitute for manual lymphatic drainage in complete decongestive therapy in the treatment of breast cancer related lymphedema. Lymphology 52.2 (2019): 82-91.

Scaglioni, Mario F., et al. Comprehensive review of vascularized lymph node transfers for lymphedema: outcomes and complications. Microsurgery 38.2 (2018): 222-229.

Schaverien, Mark V., et al. Liposuction treatment of lymphedema. Seminars in Plastic Surgery 32.1 (2018): 42-47.

Scheer, Robyn. Compression garments for managing lymphoedema. Journal of Lymphoedema 12.1 (2017): 39-45.

Schmitz, Kathryn H., et al. Physical activity and lymphedema (the PAL trial): assessing the safety of progressive strength training in breast cancer survivors. Contemporary Clinical Trials 30 (2009a): 233-245.

Schmitz, Kathryn H., et al. Weight lifting in women with breast-cancer –related lymphedema. New England Journal of Medicine 361.7 (2009b): 664-673.

Schmitz, Kathryn H., et al. Weight lifting for women at risk for breast cancer–related lymphedema: a randomized trial. JAMA 304.24 (2010): 2699-2705.

Schmitz, Kathryn H., et al. Effect of home-based exercise and weight loss programs on breast cancer–related lymphedema outcomes among overweight breast cancer survivors: the WISER Survivor randomized clinical trial. JAMA Oncology 5.11 (2019): 1605-1613.

Sen, Yuka, et al. Breast cancer-related lymphedema: differentiating fat from fluid using magnetic resonance imaging segmentation. Lymphatic Research and Biology 16.1 (2018): 20-27.

Shimbo, Keisuke, et al. Comparative study of conservative treatment and lymphaticovenular anastomosis with compression therapy for early-stage breast cancer-related lymphoedema. Journal of Plastic, Reconstructive & Aesthetic Surgery 88 (2024): 390-396.

Showalter, Shayna L., et al. Lifestyle risk factors associated with arm swelling among women with breast cancer. Annals of Surgical Oncology 20 (2013): 842-849.

Singh, Benjamin, et al. Effects of compression on lymphoedema during resistance exercise in women with breast cancer-related lymphoedema: a randomised, cross-over trial. Lymphology 48.2 (2015): 80-92.

Soga, Masashi, et al. Gardening is beneficial for health: a meta-analysis. Preventive Medicine Reports 5 (2017): 92-99.

Soran, Atilla, et al. The importance of detection of subclinical lymphedema for the prevention of breast cancer-related clinical lymphedema after axillary lymph node dissection: a prospective observational study. Lymphatic Research and Biology 12.4 (2014): 289-294.

Stemmer, Robert. A clinical symptom for the early and differential diagnosis of lymphedema. Vasa 5.3 (1976): 261-262.

Suami, Hiroo, et al. Patterns of lymphatic drainage after axillary node dissection impact arm lymphoedema severity: a review of animal and clinical imaging studies. Surgical Oncology 27.4 (2018): 743-750.

Taylor, Richard, et al. Reliability and validity of arm volume measurements for assessment of lymphedema. Physical Therapy 86.2 (2006): 205-214.

Thomas, Kim S., et al. Penicillin to prevent recurrent leg cellulitis. New England Journal of Medicine 368.18 (2013): 1695-1703.

Todd, Marie. Selecting compression hosiery. British Journal of Nursing 24.4 (2015): 210-212.

Torres Lacomba, María, et al. Axillary web syndrome after axillary dissection in breast cancer: a prospective study. Breast Cancer Research and Treatment 117 (2009): 625-630.

US Medical Compression Alliance [**USMCA**]. US medical compression consensus document. Lymphedema Treatment Act (2018): https://usmedicalcompressionalliance.com/usmca-consensus-document

Uzkeser, Hulya, et al. Efficacy of manual lymphatic drainage and intermittent pneumatic compression pump use in the treatment of lymphedema after mastectomy: a randomized controlled trial. Breast Cancer 22.3 (2015): 300-307.

Vargo, Mary, et al. Current diagnostic and quantitative techniques in the field of lymphedema management: a critical review. Medical Oncology 41.10 (2024): 241.

Verbelen, Hanne, et al. Breast edema in breast cancer patients following breast-conserving surgery and radiotherapy: a systematic review. Breast Cancer Research and Treatment 147 (2014): 463-471.

Vignes, S., et al. Complications of autologous lymph-node transplantation for limb lymphoedema. European Journal of Vascular and Endovascular Surgery 45.5 (2013): 516-520.

Vignes, Stéphane, et al. Cellulitis risk factors for patients with primary or secondary lymphedema. Journal of Vascular Surgery: Venous and Lymphatic Disorders 10.1 (2022): 179-185.

Walker, James, et al. A systematic review of pharmacologic and cell-based therapies for treatment of lymphedema (2010-2021). Journal of Vascular Surgery: Venous and Lymphatic Disorders 10.4 (2022): 966-975.

Webb, Elizabeth, et al. Compression therapy to prevent recurrent cellulitis of the leg. New England Journal of Medicine 383.7 (2020): 630-639.

Winch, Caleb J., et al. Sexual concerns of women diagnosed with breast cancer-related lymphedema. Supportive Care in Cancer 23.12 (2015): 3481-3491.

Yang, Fu-An, et al. Effect of kinesiology taping on breast cancer-related lymphedema: a systematic review and meta-analysis of randomized controlled trials. Clinical Breast Cancer 24.6 (2024): 541-551.

Yeung, W. M., et al. A systematic review of axillary web syndrome (AWS). Journal of Cancer Survivorship 9 (2015): 576-598.

Young-Afat, Danny A., et al. Breast edema following breast-conserving surgery and radiotherapy: patient-reported prevalence, determinants, and effect on health-related quality of life. JNCI Cancer Spectrum 3.2 (2019).

INDEX

A

Air travel, 119, 127–129
ALERT Centre, 41, 43–46, 56, 58, 60, 97, 99–102, 104, 107–109, 111, 116, 119–120, 129, 155, 160
Anatomy, 15–19
- Axillary lymph nodes, 18–19, 45, 145
- Epitrochlear node, 17
- Interval lymph nodes, 17
- Lymphatic capillaries, 16
- Lymphatic vessels, 15–19
- Regional lymph nodes, 17, 119
- Supraclavicular fossa, 19, 27, 29, 32, 53
- Thoracic duct, 16, 58
- Venule, 111

Antibiotics, 22, 120, 127, 134, 136–140. *See also Yoghurt*
- Prophylactic antibiotics, 138–139

Armpit (axilla), 17–19
Australasian Lymphology Association (ALA), 138, 158, 163
Axillary radiation, 146
Axillary surgery, 27, 31, 114, 120
- Lymph node dissection, 27–30, 111, 113, 119, 148
- Sentinel node biopsy, 18, 28–29, 32, 53, 119, 147

Axillary web syndrome. *See Cording*

B

Bandaging, 55–56, 59–63, 67, 77, 86, 101
- Two-layer short-stretch, 62

Bioimpedance spectroscopy (BIS), 22, 28, 40, 42, 50–51, 53, 97, 127, 152. *See also Diagnosis of lymphoedema; L-Dex; SOZO*
Blood draws, 120, 128
Blood pressure, 121, 128
Body image, 88, 160–161
Bras, 149–150, 153
Breast oedema, 92, 133, 142, 144–155
- Clinical features, 148–149
- Compression pump, 150
- Definition, 78
- Diagnosis, 148–151
- Imaging, 150–151
- Treatment, 152–155

British Lymphology Society (BLS), 120, 137–139, 170

C

Cellulitis, 133–141
- Abscess, 135
- Bacteria, 15, 72, 74, 125, 134, 136–138, 140
- Blood tests, 120
- Prevention, 138–139
- Staphylococcus, 137, 140
- Streptococcus, 137
- Symptoms, 21, 68, 93, 101, 145
- Treatment, 137

Circumference, 35, 37, 39–41, 53, 68, 96, 112
Comfiwave, 66, 105
Complete decongestive therapy (CDT). *See Complex lymphoedema therapy (CLT)*

Complex lymphoedema therapy (CLT), 55
Components, 55
Compression pumps, 55, 154
Exercise, 64
Maintenance phase, 55, 60, 66–67, 69, 86
Manual lymphatic drainage, 45, 55–56, 58–60, 66, 68, 152
Pneumatic compression, 60, 66–69, 77, 116, 154
Reduction phase, 56, 64
Skin care, 58, 71
Compression, 60, 67, 77–89
Compression bandages, 56, 60
Compression bra, 153–154
Compression garments, 77–86
Circular vs flat-knit, 79–80
Classes (levels), 78
Custom-made garments, 83, 103
Donning (putting on), 87
Durability, 74, 80, 85
Looking after, 87–88
Ready-to-wear garments, 82
Compression pump, 60, 66–69, 77
Compression therapy, 56, 60, 77, 93, 100
Cording, 30–33, 49
Aspirin, 32, 123
Mondor's disease, 32–33

D

Deep venous thrombosis, 89
Diagnosis of lymphoedema, 44, 129. *See also Bioimpedance spectroscopy (BIS)*
Clinical examination, 35–37
Dimpling, 149
Discomfort, 22, 30, 72, 154
Infrared, 41, 43, 92, 151
L-Dex, 42, 50–53, 58, 97, 124
Moisture meter, 47, 150
Nuclear studies, 42
Perometer, 27, 41, 50
Physical examination, 42, 56
Pitting test, 25, 38, 100
SOZO, 50–52. *See also Bioimpedance spectroscopy (BIS)*
Tissue dielectric constant, 47, 150
Dicloxacillin, 137, 139
Donning (putting on), 87
Arthritis, 63, 77
Doxycycline, 94, 137, 139

E

Early detection and intervention, 49. *See also Bioimpedance spectroscopy (BIS); L-Dex; Perometry; SOZO; Stages of lymphoedema; Symptoms of lymphoedema*
Education, 55–57, 82, 97, 104, 141, 159, 166
Education and support, 55, 57
Elephantiasis, 23
Erysipelas, 133. *See also Cellulitis*
Erythromycin, 139
Examination, 35–36, 42, 56, 149
Exercise, 64
Aerobic, 112
Flexibility, 31, 64, 164
Mobility, 36, 67–68, 93, 100–101, 165
Muscle-strengthening, 64–65, 123–124
Neuropathy, 157
Yoga, 164–165

F

Fibrosis, 23, 25, 37, 55, 57, 59, 87
Flucloxacillin, 137
Fungal infections, 57, 75, 140

G

Gardening, 125
  Antihistamines, 127
Garments, 77–89
  Anti-embolism stockings, 77
  Gauntlet, 81–82, 84
  Glove, 64, 81–82, 84, 96
  Sleeve, 49, 67, 81, 84, 96, 106, 129, 142–143, 162, 166
  Velcro, 63, 83

H

Haddenham, 63, 66, 82–83, 105

I

Imaging techniques, 111
  ICG. *See Indocyanine green lymphography*
  Lymphoscintigraphy, 42–43
  Mammography, 147, 150
  MRI, 46, 100
  Ultrasound, 147, 150–152
Indentation, 23–25, 37, 100, 148–149
Indocyanine green lymphography, 43, 45, 111, 116, 151
  Dermal backflow, 43–45, 59–60, 151–152
Inflammation, 23–24, 30–32, 71–72, 91, 95, 133–134, 136
Injection, 42, 122, 151
Insect bite. *See Precautions*
Intravenous, 129, 137

K

Kinesiology taping, 93, 154–155

L

L-Dex, 42, 50–53, 58, 97, 124. *See also Bioimpedance spectroscopy (BIS)*
Laser therapy, 32, 91–92, 116. *See also Photobiomodulation (laser)*
  Low-level laser therapy, 91
  MLS, 92
LE&RN Centers of Excellence, 174
Liposuction, 99–105
  Adipose tissue, 23–24
Lumpectomy, 96, 106, 116, 145
Lymph node transfer, 114–115, 117 *See also Surgery for lymphoedema*
Lymphangion, 17
Lymphangitis, 71, 133
Lymphatic fluid, 22–24, 30, 40, 44–46, 50, 58–60, 64–65, 67, 73, 78, 93–95, 100, 114, 149–151
Lymphoedema incidence, 27–29, 146–147
Lymphorrhoea, 71, 117
Lymphovenous anastomosis (LVA), 111–112, 114, 116–117, 155. *See also Surgery for lymphoedema*

M

Magnetic resonance imaging, 46, 100
Manual lymphatic drainage, 45, 55–56, 58–60, 66, 68, 152
Moisturisers, 56, 73–74, 85
Monitoring for lymphoedema, 41, 50. *See also Bioimpedance spectroscopy (BIS); L-Dex*

N

Night-time garments, 66–67, 85–86
Numbness, 49, 64, 103, 117
Nutrition, 57

O

Obesity, 133

P

Perometry, 27, 41, 50
PET-CT scan, 89
Photobiomodulation (laser), 91–92
Pitting, 22–25, 37–38, 49, 100
Pneumatic compression, 60, 66–69, 77, 116, 154
Postoperative, 50, 101–103, 105, 112
Precautions, 65, 71, 118–120, 125–127, 129
- Air travel, 119, 127–129
- Blood draws, 120, 128
- Blood pressure, 121, 128
- Climate, 124, 128
- Clotting, 30, 32
- Exercise, 65
- Gardening, 125
- Heat, 125, 128
- Injections, 42, 119–120, 128, 151
- Insect repellent, 71, 126, 128

PREVENT study, 28–29, 50–51, 119
Prevention, 22, 29, 55, 66, 72, 74, 120, 127, 129–130, 132, 140
Primary lymphoedema, 36
Prophylactic antibiotics, 138–139

Q

Quality of life, 102, 124–125, 148, 157–161

R

Randomised controlled trial, 86, 94, 96, 113, 123–124, 139–140, 152, 165
Risk factors for lymphoedema, 26–27, 29, 119, 129. *See also Cellulitis; Cording*
- Chemotherapy, 27–29, 53
- Lymph node dissection, 27–30, 111, 113, 119, 148
- Radiation therapy, 27–29, 32, 53
- Taxanes, 27, 119

Risk reduction, 128, 130

S

Scarring, 21, 23, 25, 37, 49
Secondary lymphoedema, 36, 107
Self-management, 55
- Acupuncture, 95–96, 164
- Alcohol, 35, 122
- BMI, 27, 29, 139, 147
- Body image, 88, 160–161
- Counselling, 159–160
- Diabetes, 35, 57–58, 88, 133
- Emotional, 36, 57, 143, 156, 160–161, 163–165
- Footwear, 64
- Intimacy, 88, 160
- Sauna, 125
- Sunscreen, 125–126, 128
- Weight, 29, 40, 53, 58, 77, 86, 95, 101, 108, 123–124, 149, 153
- Yoga, 164–165

Sequential intermittent pneumatic compression (SIPC), 55, 60, 66–69, 77, 154
Skin care, 71–75
- Acidic, 73–74
- Antibacterial cream, 74, 126

Antifungal cream, 75, 140
Betadine, 122, 140–141
Coconut oil, 74
Dishwashing, 73
Disinfectants, 74
Hibiclens, 141
Hydration, 51, 126
Nail care, 58
Scaliness, 75
SOZO, 50–52. *See also Bioimpedance spectroscopy (BIS)*
Stages of lymphoedema, 23–24, 37. *See also Fibrosis*
Surgery for lymphoedema, 99–109, 111–117
Bruising, 103, 117, 123
Complications, 32, 36, 41, 55, 71, 95, 102–103, 105, 115, 117, 126
Liposuction, 24, 86, 98–106, 108–109, 138, 163–164
Lymph node transfer, 114–115, 117
Lymphatic microsurgery, 110–111, 115, 117, 138, 155
Lymphovenous anastomosis (LVA), 111–112, 114, 116–117, 155
Symptoms of lymphoedema, 21

T

Tests for lymphoedema, 39
Tinea, 75, 133
Tissue dielectric constant, 47, 150
Treatment of lymphoedema (other), 91, 94–95
Benzopyrones, 94–95
Corticosteroids, 95
Diuretics, 94
Experimental, 35, 114
Ketoprofen, 94–95

V

Vaccination, 122–123
Vascularised lymph node transfer. *See Lymph node transfer* 114–115, 117
Venepuncture. *See Blood draws* 120, 128

Y

Yoga, 164–165
Yoghurt, 138